T0228075

Principles and Practicalities of ENT

Principles and Practicalities of ENT is a resource allowing both students and doctors of all levels to approach common clinical scenarios encountered in ENT with confidence. Each section will take you through how to prepare for patients, key points in the history and examination and how best to investigate and manage a wide variety of common ENT presentations and conditions. The material is structured to provide an easy reference, including red flag and primary care sections to enable readers to know what to look out for when considering referrals. Therefore, in addition to being a revision tool for medical students, doctors pursuing MRCS (ENT) examinations and higher surgical training in ENT, this book can also serve as a useful aid for primary care physicians in their everyday diagnostics and referral practices.

Principles and Practicalities of ENT

How to approach common clinical scenarios

Keshav K. Gupta
Divya Vatish
Karan Jolly
Duncan Bowyer

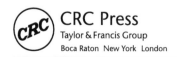

CRC Press
Taylor & Francis Group
Boca Raton New York London

CRC Press is an imprint of the
Taylor & Francis Group, an **informa** business

First edition published 2023
by CRC Press
6000 Broken Sound Parkway NW, Suite 300, Boca Raton, FL 33487-2742

and by CRC Press
4 Park Square, Milton Park, Abingdon, Oxon, OX14 4RN

CRC Press is an imprint of Taylor & Francis Group, LLC

© 2023 Taylor & Francis Group, LLC

ISBN: 9781032209012 (hbk)
ISBN: 9781032207285 (pbk)
ISBN: 9781003265917 (ebk)

DOI: 10.1201/b23238

Typeset in Goudy Oldstyle Std
by KnowledgeWorks Global Ltd.

This book is dedicated to Professor Ravindra K. Dhir OBE

Contents

Acknowledgment

We would like to thank Mrs Krupali Gupta, Mr Zahir Mughal and Dr Elizabeth Moor for their artistic skills in recreating figures. We would also like to thank Mr Richard Irving and Mr Charlie Huins for their help with providing clinical photographs.

Author biographies

Mr. Keshav K. Gupta, MBBS BSc (Hons) MRCS (ENT), is an ENT specialty registrar in the West Midlands Deanery, UK, who secured a competitive training post at national selection in 2021, on his first attempt. He graduated from Imperial College London in 2017 with multiple prizes and distinctions. Keshav has been heavily involved in teaching at undergraduate and postgraduate levels and has designed and implemented many teaching courses. He has published book chapters and more than 30 papers in peer-reviewed journals. Keshav has presented his work at national and international conferences and won multiple research, presentation and surgical simulation prizes.

Dr. Divya Vatish, MBBS BSc (Hons) DRCOG MRCGP, is a qualified GP who graduated in 2017 from Barts and the London School of Medicine and Dentistry. Divya has a keen interest in teaching, having secured a first class honours in her BSc in Medical Education. She also currently works as a Technology Enhanced Learning Fellow with Health Education West Midlands, helping to develop virtual and blended learning platforms for GP trainees.

Mr. Karan Jolly, MBChB DOHNS FRCS (ORL-HNS), is a consultant ENT surgeon with a special interest in rhinology and anterior skull base surgery having recently completed training in the UK and Canada. Karan has been actively involved in research over his training years with over 40 peer-reviewed publications, book chapter publications and national awards including the inaugural Sir Cecil Wakeley Medal. He is also very actively involved in training and education, being a faculty member on several courses and co-authoring on a FRCS VIVA revision book.

Mr. Duncan Bowyer, BSc (Hons) MBBS DOHNS FRCS (ORL-HNS) FFSTEd, is a consultant ENT surgeon at Shrewsbury & Telford Hospital NHS Trust (UK). Alongside his clinical practice, he has a varied medical education portfolio; he is an undergraduate lecturer at Keele Medical School, training programme director for Otolaryngology Higher Surgical Training in the West Midlands, examiner for the DOHNS examination, interviewer for Otolaryngology National Selection, course director and faculty on numerous skills courses, and a fellow of the Faculty of Surgical Trainers at RCS Edinburgh.

List of abbreviations

AABR	automated auditory brainstem response test
AC	air conduction
ALS	advanced life support
AMPLE	allergies, medications, past medical history, last meal timing
AOAE	automated otoacoustic emissions test
AOM	acute otitis media
APLS	advanced paediatric life support
ARS	acute rhinosinusitis
ATLS	advanced trauma life support
AV	arteriovenous
BAHA	bone anchored hearing aid
BC	bone conduction
BCHI	bone conducting hearing implant
BIPP	bismuth iodoform paraffin paste
BLS	basic life support
BPPV	benign positional paroxysmal vertigo
BSIT	Brief Smell Identification Test
BTA	British Thyroid Association
BTE	behind the ear (hearing aid)
CBT	cognitive behavioural therapy
CCRCT	Connecticut Chemosensory Clinical Research Centre orthonasal olfactory Test
CEA	carcinoembryonic antigen
CHL	conductive hearing loss
CICV	"can't intubate, can't ventilate" scenario
CMV	cytomegalovirus
CN	cranial nerve
COVID-19	severe acute respiratory syndrome coronavirus 2 (2019 novel coronavirus)
CO_2	carbon dioxide
CPAP	continuous positive airway pressure
CPR	cardiopulmonary resuscitation
CROS	contralateral routing of sound (hearing aid)
CRP	C-reactive protein
CRS	chronic rhinosinusitis
CSF	cerebrospinal fluid
CT	computed tomography
CXR	chest X-ray
dB	decibels
EAC	external auditory canal
EBV	Epstein–Barr virus
ED	emergency department
ENT	ear, nose and throat
EPI	echo planar imaging
ESR	erythrocyte sedimentation rate
EUA	examination under anaesthesia

FB	foreign body
FBC	full blood count
FESS	functional endoscopic sinus surgery
FNAC	fine needle aspiration cytology
FNE	flexible nasoendoscopy
FONA	front of neck access
Fr	French
FSH	follicle stimulating hormone
g	gram
GA	general anaesthetic
GABA	gamma-aminobutyric acid
GCS	Glasgow Coma Score
GI	gastrointestinal
GORD	gastro-oesophageal reflux disease
GP	general practitioner
GRBAS	global score, roughness, breathiness, asthenia, strain
HDU	high dependency unit
HFNC	high-flow nasal cannula
HINTS	head impulse test, nystagmus, test of skew
HIV	human immunodeficiency virus
HPV	human papillomavirus
IAM	internal acoustic meatus
ICU	intensive care unit
INR	international normalised ratio
IV	intravenous
kg	kilogram
LA	local anaesthetic
LFT	liver function test
LH	luteinising hormones
LPR	laryngopharyngeal reflux
mc&s	microscopy, sensitivity and culture
MDT	multidisciplinary team
MEN	multiple endocrine neoplasia
mg	milligram
mL	millilitres
mmHg	millimetres of mercury
MRI	magnetic resonance imaging
MTC	medullary thyroid carcinoma
MUA	manipulation under anaesthesia
NBM	nil by mouth
NF	neruofibromatosis
NGT	nasogastric tube
NHSP	newborn hearing screening programme
NICU	neonatal intensive care unit
NSAID	non-steroidal anti-inflammatory drug
OE	otitis externa
OGD	oesophagogastroduododenoscopy
OM	otitis media
OME	otitis media with effusion (glue ear)

OMFS	oral maxillofacial surgery
OSA	obstructive sleep apnoea
PDMS	polydimethylsiloxane
PET	positron emission tomography
PICC	peripherally inserted central catheter
PICU	paediatric intensive care unit
PNS	post-nasal space
PPI	proton pump inhibitor
PTA	pure-tone audiometry
PTB	post-tonsillectomy bleed
RAPD	relative afferent pupillary defect
RAST	radioallergosorbent test
SCC	squamous cell carcinoma
SCM	sternocleidomastoid muscle
SLT	speech and language therapy
SNHL	sensorineural hearing loss
SNOT-22	sinonasal outcome test
SOB	shortness of breath
SSCD	superior semicircular canal dehiscence
SSNHL	sudden sensorineural hearing loss
TB	tuberculosis
TFT	thyroid function test
TLM	transoral laser microsurgery
TM	tympanic membrane
TMJ	temporomandibular joint
TNM	tumour, node, metastasis staging classification
TOD	Teacher of the Deaf
TORS	transoral robotic surgery
TPN	total parenteral nutrition
TSH	thyroid stimulating hormone
U&Es	urea and electrolytes
UPSIT	University of Pennsylvania Smell Identification Test
URTI	upper respiratory tract infection
US	ultrasound
USS	ultrasound scan
VAS	visual analogue scale
VBG	venous blood gas
VEMP	vestibular evoked myogenic potential testing
VHI	Voice Handicap Index
VKG	videokymography
VLS	videolaryngostroboscopy
VOR	vestibulo-ocular reflex
VRA	visually reinforced audiometry
XR	X-ray

Section I

Emergency

Otology

Chapter 1

Mastoiditis

Background

Acute mastoiditis is an inflammatory process of the mastoid air cell system that is usually a sequela of acute otitis media (AOM). The condition is more common in males and has a peak incidence of 1–3 years. The causative organisms are similar to those of bacterial AOM, with *Strep. pneumoniae, Strep. pyogenes, Haemophilus influenzae, Staph. aureus* and *Pseudomonas aeruginosa* being the most common. In severe cases of AOM, mucosal oedema may block the communication between the middle ear and mastoid, trapping infected secretions in the mastoid. The resulting increased pressure causes localised bony necrosis that results in coalescent mastoiditis. Further spread of the infection through the mastoid cortex causes postauricular cellulitis and eventually a subperiosteal abscess. It is important to diagnose and treat acute mastoiditis early to prevent further progression. This can include intracranial spread, resulting in meningitis, intracranial abscesses, otic hydrocephalus and venous sinus thrombosis. Other, rarer sequelae include facial paralysis, acute petrositis and labyrinthitis.

Potential areas for deterioration

C – risk of septic shock
D – risk of intracranial sepsis

Preparation and equipment

- This is an ENT emergency, and the patient must be seen urgently.
- Involve members of the MDT early (paediatrics, microbiology).
- Attend the patient with an otoscope.

History

Symptoms

- Onset, timing and duration
- Laterality
- Radiation of pain
- Better or worse
- Exacerbating or relieving factors
- Previous treatments and their effects
- Previous episodes (especially requiring hospital admission)

DOI: 10.1201/b23238-3

Systems

- Ear – otalgia, otorrhoea, tinnitus, vertigo, hearing loss, facial weakness
- Intracranial – nausea, vomiting, headache, loss of consciousness, seizures, rashes, features of meningism
- Change in child's behaviour – poor feeding, irritability, clumsiness
- Systemic features – fever, nausea, vomiting

Red flags/risk factors

- Immunocompromise
- Rapid clinical deterioration
- Features of intracranial involvement

AMPLE

- Allergies, regular/recent medications, other relevant past medical history, time of last meal
- Paediatrics – antenatal and obstetric complications, developmental history and immunisation status

Examination

- General inspection – unwell looking child, toxic appearance
- Ear – signs of AOM (redness and bulging of the tympanic membrane [TM])
- Mastoid process – tender, erythematous, boggy swelling, loss of postauricular sulcus, displacement of pinna antero-inferiorly (Figure 1.1)
- Neurological – Glasgow Coma Score (GCS), cranial nerve assessment, signs of meningism (nuchal rigidity, non-blanching rash, Kernig's sign, Brudzinski's sign)
- Full set of observations – assess for signs of sepsis (fever, tachycardia, hypotension, tachypnoea)

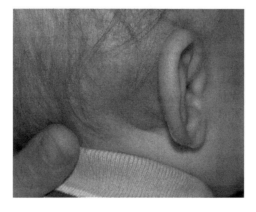

Figure 1.1 Clinical photograph of patient with mastoiditis. (Courtesy of Mr. Richard Irving.)

Management

The principle of management in patients with mastoiditis is to clear the infection, with antimicrobial therapy and/or surgical intervention. Microbiology samples, blood tests and imaging are useful adjuncts to help guide management.

Bedside investigations

- Ear swab – mc&s
- Blood tests – FBC, U&Es, CRP, venous blood gas (VBG) with lactate, blood cultures

Imaging

- CT temporal bones – useful to confirm diagnosis (Figure 1.2)
  - Demineralisation/coalescence of mastoid air cells, opaque mastoid and middle ear
  - Overlying soft tissue thickening or subperiosteal abscess
- CT brain with contrast – assessing for intracranial complications
  - Extradural/subdural/brain abscess
  - Sigmoid sinus thrombosis
- MRI brain has higher sensitivity than CT for intracranial complications

Medical

- IV antibiotics are administered to cover common organisms.
- Convert to oral antibiotics once afebrile for 48 hours and there are signs of resolving infection.
- Analgesia.

Surgical

- Keep the patient nil by mouth (NBM).
- Informed consent of the patient by explaining benefits, risks and alternatives.

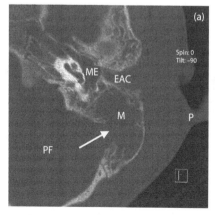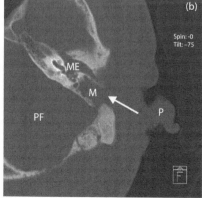

Figure 1.2 Axial CT of the temporal bone in acute mastoiditis: (a) With erosion of sigmoid sinus plate (arrow); (b) Cortical erosion (arrow) with subperiosteal abscess. (*Abbreviations:* P: pinna, M: mastoid, EAC: external auditory canal, ME: middle ear, PF: posterior fossa.)

- Surgical intervention is indicated when radiological evidence of abscess, failure to respond to IV antibiotic therapy after 24–48 hours and/or if concerns regarding intracranial extension.
- Incision and drainage of subperiosteal abscess.
- Cortical mastoidectomy.
- Myringotomy and ventilation tube insertion.
- Neurosurgical involvement for intracranial complications.

Discharge and follow-up

- Patients can be discharged once there is resolution of infection.
- Complete full course of oral antibiotics.
- Follow-up may involve a combination of specialties (ENT, paediatrics, neurosurgery).

RED FLAGS

- Signs and symptoms of intracranial extension or evidence on imaging
- Failure to response to IV antibiotics within 24–48 hours

WHEN TO REFER FROM PRIMARY CARE

To ED
- Signs of shock (tachycardia, high pyrexia, low blood pressure)
- Failure to respond to community-prescribed oral antibiotics
- Signs of mastoiditis on examination

Chapter 2

Necrotising otitis externa

Background

Necrotising otitis externa (NOE) is an uncommon but dangerous progression of disease in (typically immunocompromised) patients with otitis externa (OE). Sometimes referred to as malignant OE, it is diagnosed when OE extends beyond the ear canal into the temporal bone and can progress to skull base osteomyelitis. Inflammatory soft-tissue thickening is typically seen in the floor of external ear canal at the osseocartilaginous junction. There may also be an extension into the temporomandibular joint (TMJ) and middle ear. The condition is most common in elderly male diabetics with poor glycaemic control. The most common causative organism is *Pseudomonas aeruginosa*. The key feature in patients with NOE is unremitting, deep-seated otalgia that interferes with sleep and activities of daily living. Patients have often had multiple courses of antibiotic therapy. Pain is out of proportion to the clinical signs, and there is a potential risk of developing facial nerve palsy and other cranial neuropathies.

Potential areas for deterioration

D – risk of intracranial extension

Preparation and equipment

- The patient may be referred to the emergency department (ED) or to a clinic.
- See the patient with an otoscope or microscope.

History

Symptoms

- Onset, timing and duration
- Laterality
- Radiation of pain
- Previous episodes including previous treatments and their effects
- Exacerbating and relieving factors
- Effect on activities of daily living and quality of life

DOI: 10.1201/b23238-4

Systems

- Ear – otorrhoea, tinnitus, vertigo, hearing loss, facial weakness
- Neurological – headaches, syncope, seizures, loss of consciousness, vomiting
- Systemic – fever

Red flags/risk factors

- Age >50 years
- States of immunocompromise and prior malignancy
- Poor diabetic control and HbA1c
- Smokers
- Deep-seated otalgia worse at night
- Granulations from inferior external auditory canal (EAC)
- Prior failed treatment
- Features of intracranial and cranial nerve involvement

AMPLE

- Allergies, regular/recent medications, other relevant past medical history, time of last meal

Examination

- Ear – signs of OE with debris in an erythematous canal, granulation tissue/polyps on inferior canal wall (Figure 2.1)
- Neurological – GCS, upper and lower limb examination
- Cranial nerves – especially those at high risk (facial and lower cranial nerves, glossopharyngeal, vagus, accessory, hypoglossal)
- Full set of observations – assess for signs of sepsis (fever, tachycardia, hypotension, tachypnoea)

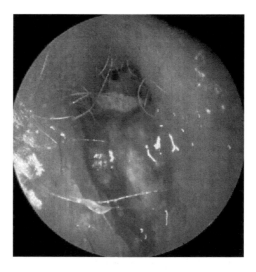

Figure 2.1 Clinical photograph of ear canal polyp in NOE.

Management

The principle of management in patients with NOE is to clear the infection and reverse any contributing host factors (e.g. tight glycaemic control). This usually requires a prolonged course of systemic antibiotics (at least 6–8 weeks) with regular aural toilet. The use of microbiology swabs, biopsies, bloods tests and imaging are useful adjuncts to help guide management and monitor response to treatment.

Bedside investigations

- Ear swab – mc&s
- Biopsy – of any polyps/granulation tissue
- Cautery – silver nitrate cautery can help shrink large polyps
- Bloods – FBC, U&Es, ESR, CRP, blood cultures
- PTA – formal hearing test as a baseline before commencing treatment

Imaging

- CT temporal bones – presence of bony erosion
- MRI head with contrast – assess the extent of soft tissue involvement and intracranial involvement
- Radionucleotide scans
  - Technetium – diagnosis (enhances osteoblast and osteoclast activity)
  - Indium or gallium scintigraphy – monitoring response to treatment (enhances white cell activity)

Medical

- Long-term IV antibiotics, usually for 6–8 weeks.
- Low-risk patients can be managed on an outpatient basis with oral ciprofloxacin and regular review.
- Regular aural toilet and topical antibiotics (e.g. ciprofloxacin) to the affected ear.
- Analgesia.
- Optimise glycaemic control, often with input from diabetic team.
- Regular monitoring of clinical progression: otalgia, ear examination, observations, inflammatory markers (ESR is more useful than CRP).

Adjunct

- Speech and Language Therapy (SLT) input for lower cranial nerve palsies if affecting speech/swallowing.
- Facial nerve palsy management (e.g. ophthalmology involvement).
- Surgical debridement is rarely used.
- Hyperbaric oxygen may play a role if locally available.

Discharge and follow-up

- Long-term IV antibiotic therapy can be continued in the community with a PICC line.
- IV antibiotics are generally recommended to continue for 4–6 weeks after the patient is pain-free.
- Multidisciplinary team (MDT) involvement (ENT, infectious disease/microbiology, radiology, SLT, diabetic team).
- Patients require regular outpatient monitoring during treatment.

RED FLAGS

- Unremitting, deep-seated otalgia
- Not responding to first-line antimicrobial therapy
- Elderly male diabetic patients
- Poor diabetic control
- Immunocompromise
- Symptoms or signs of cranial neuropathy or intracranial extension

WHEN TO REFER FROM PRIMARY CARE

To ED

- Septic patient
- Intracranial involvement
- Outpatient CT scan results showing evidence of NOE
- High clinical suspicion of NOE

To emergency clinic

- Patients with signs and symptoms of OE who also have:
    - not responded to 2 or more course of appropriate topical antibiotic therapy
    - an inflamed, erythematous, stenosed ear canal that may require a wick
    - obstructive debris that may require microsuction

Chapter 3

Sudden sensorineural hearing loss

Background

Sudden sensorineural hearing loss (SSNHL) is defined as sensorineural hearing loss of 30 dB or more over three continuous audiometric frequencies occurring in less than 72 hours. The majority of patients presenting with SSNHL have no identifiable cause (idiopathic). It is important to consider other causes of sudden hearing loss (Table 3.1). Early identification and management of patients with SSNHL result in improved long-term hearing outcomes. Optimal acute management is controversial, although the widely accepted treatment of SSNHL is with prompt use of high-dose corticosteroids. These may be administered orally or through intratympanic injection. Corticosteroids are thought to reduce inflammation and oedema in the inner ear. Even patients who receive early corticosteroid therapy may not regain full hearing, and recovery may take many months. It is important to counsel patients regarding this. Poor prognostic factors for hearing recovery include age >60 years, severe/ profound hearing losses, a flat or downsloping hearing pattern on pure tone audiometry (PTA), associated vertigo and no hearing recovery in the first few weeks.

Preparation and equipment

- This patient may be referred to ED or to a clinic.
- See the patient with an otoscope and facilities for PTA and tympanometry.

History

Symptoms

- Onset, timing and duration.
- Laterality.
- What were they doing at the time and how did they notice it?
- Better or worse.
- Previous episodes including previous treatments and their effects.
- Exposure to loud noise.
- Trauma.

Systems

- Ear – otalgia, otorrhoea, tinnitus, vertigo, facial weakness
- Neurological – slurred speech, limb weakness
- Autoimmune – fevers, rash, ulcers, myalgia, joint pain, visual disturbance, malaise, recurrent thrombosis, dry mucous membranes, weight loss

DOI: 10.1201/b23238-5

Table 3.1 Causes of sudden hearing loss

Common causes	Idiopathic, trauma, noise-induced
Otological	TM perforation, AOM, OE
Neurological	Stroke
Autoimmune	Lupus, antiphospholipid syndrome, polyarteritis nodosa, Sjögren's syndrome, rheumatoid arthritis, sarcoid
Infection	Measles, mumps, meningitis
Inflammation	Labyrinthitis
Malignancy	Vestibular schwannoma, meningioma

Past medical history

- Autoimmune disease (as in Table 3.1)
- Previous otological history and surgery

Drug history

- Allergies
- Ototoxic drugs – salicylates, loop diuretics, NSAIDs, aminoglycosides

Social history

- Smoking, alcohol status
- Performance status
- Impact on quality of life, activities of daily living and hobbies

Examination

- Assess for functional signs of hearing loss – change in speech, difficulty in hearing conversation
- Otoscopy – evidence of OE, AOM, TM perforation
- Cranial nerves (especially facial nerve)
- Neurology – gait, upper and lower limb examination
- Hearing – tuning fork, free-field hearing test

Management

The principle of management in patients presenting with SSNHL is to try and restore as much hearing function as possible. The mainstay of treatment for sudden hearing loss is corticosteroids, either oral or intratympanic.

Bedside investigations

- Hearing tests – PTA, tympanometry.
- Blood tests are required only if suspecting an undiagnosed autoimmune condition – FBC, U&Es, ESR, antinuclear antibodies (ANA), anticardiolipin antibodies, lupus anticoagulant, antineutrophil cytoplasmic antibodies (ANCA).

Imaging

- MRI internal acoustic meatus usually performed in patients with audiometrically confirmed SSNHL (routine outpatient)

Medical

- Commence oral corticosteroids (prednisolone) after discussing the risks and benefits with the patient.
- Oral prednisolone 1 mg/kg (max 60 mg) for 7 days then tapered by 10 mg a day.
- Consider dual therapy with intratympanic corticosteroids in cases with poor prognosis.
- Rate of spontaneous hearing recovery varies between 30% and 65% – this may be doubled with corticosteroid therapy.
- Consider emergency hearing aid provision if required (only hearing/better hearing ear affected).
- Counsel the patient that hearing may only partially recover or never recover.

Discharge and follow-up

- Patients with SSNHL do not need to routinely be admitted.
- Repeat PTA after completion of corticosteroid course.
- Consider salvage intratympanic corticosteroids if no improvement.

RISKS OF ORAL CORTICOSTEROIDS

- Gastrointestinal – nausea, vomiting, reflux, ulcer, change in appetite, weight gain
- Musculoskeletal – muscle weakness, osteoporosis, avascular necrosis of femoral head
- Visual – blurred vision
- Mood – nervousness, restlessness, difficulty sleeping, altered mood
- Immunosuppression
- Swollen face (moon face)
- Ecchymosis
- Hyperglycaemia and worsening of diabetic control if diabetic
- Raised blood pressure

WHEN TO REFER FROM PRIMARY CARE

- Any patient suffering from suspected SSNHL should be referred to local ENT team and oral corticosteroids should be commenced
- ENT will arrange a review for audiometric confirmation of diagnosis, +/– further investigations depending on the scenario

Chapter 4

Temporal bone trauma

Background

The temporal bone contains important structures, including the facial nerve, vestibulocochlear nerve and middle and inner ear structures (otic capsule – cochlea, vestibule and semi-circular canals). Damage to any of these or adjacent structures (including glossopharyngeal, vagus and accessory nerves, internal carotid artery and sigmoid sinus) carries significant risks of morbidity and mortality. The temporal bone is very dense and, therefore, requires significant direct force to fracture. Patients with temporal bone trauma have, therefore, usually been involved in high-impact trauma and are likely to present as part of a polytrauma scenario. Fractures of the temporal bone were historically classified as longitudinal, transverse or mixed, depending on the fracture line directionality relative to the long axis of the temporal bone. More recently, this has been reclassified into a more clinically useful system: Otic capsule violating or otic capsule sparing. This system better predicts clinical outcomes, with otic capsule violating fractures more commonly associated with hearing loss (either conductive or sensorineural), facial nerve palsy and cerebrospinal fluid (CSF) leaks.

ENT COMPLICATIONS OF TEMPORAL BONE FRACTURE

- Conductive hearing loss – ossicular chain disruption, TM perforation
- Sensorineural hearing loss – damage to cochlea
- Dead ear – irreversible damage to cochlea
- Vertigo and tinnitus – damage to cochlea/vestibular system
- Facial nerve palsy – damage to the nerve as it travels through the temporal bone
- CSF leak with subsequent risk of meningitis – damage to skull base and dura

Potential areas for deterioration

D – risk of disability through neurosurgical sequelae of a high-impact trauma scenario

Preparation and equipment

- This is an ENT emergency, and the patient must be seen promptly.
- ENT may be asked to attend as a part of the formal trauma team in the event of polytrauma; a full ENT assessment is important in an advanced trauma life support (ATLS) approach:
  - The team should attend early to introduce themselves, assign roles and receive handover from the pre-hospital team if the patient is brought in by an ambulance.

DOI: 10.1201/b23238-6

- Ensure the patient is assessed in accordance with the ATLS protocol with a primary survey.
- Deal with any other potential injuries in order of priority according to trauma scenario.

History

Events

- Preceding events
- Type of events – road traffic accident, assault
- Post-event – blood loss, loss of consciousness, seizure, amnesia

Systems

- Ear – otalgia, otorrhoea (bloody, clear), tinnitus, vertigo, hearing loss, facial weakness
- Nose – nasal trauma – deviation, epistaxis, clear rhinorrhoea
- Neurological – headaches, syncope, seizures, loss of consciousness, vomiting

Red flags/risk factors

- High-impact trauma
- Signs and symptoms of hearing loss, facial nerve palsy, CSF leak, severe vertigo

AMPLE

- Allergies, regular/recent medications, other relevant past medical history, time of last meal

Examination

- General signs of temporal bone fracture – battle sign (postauricular ecchymosis), raccoon eyes (periorbital ecchymosis)
- Otoscopy – bloody otorrhoea, CSF otorrhoea, hemotympanum, TM perforation, visible EAC fracture line
- Nose – deviation, septal haematoma, epistaxis, CSF rhinorrhoea
- Cranial nerves (especially facial nerve)
- Hearing – tuning fork, free-field hearing test
- Full set of observations

Management

The principle of managing patients with temporal bone trauma is to identify and treat any damage to temporal bone structures. Subsequent management may be done as an inpatient or outpatient depending on the presentation.

Bedside investigations

- Ear/nasal discharge – send for tau protein/beta-2 transferrin analysis to confirm CSF
- Blood tests – FBC, U&Es, coagulation profile, group and save/crossmatch as part of the trauma scenario
- Inpatient PTA and tympanogram if possible

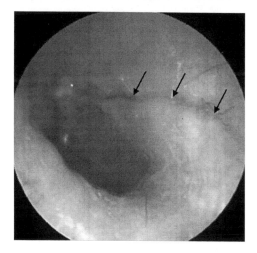

Figure 4.1 Otoendoscopic photograph of temporal bone fracture involving bony ear canal (arrows).

Imaging

- CT traumogram will likely be conducted as part of the trauma scenario
- CT head confirms temporal bone fracture – fracture line, pneumocranium, opacification within middle ear cleft
- CT temporal bones – otic capsule violating or sparing (Figure 4.1)
  - Ossicular discontinuity
  - Otic capsule damage
  - Facial nerve dehiscence
  - CSF leak
  - Perilymph fistula
- MRI brain – localise CSF leak

General

- Consider tetanus booster and tranexamic acid, if indicated
- Analgesia

CSF leak

- Aim to prevent or treat meningitis
- Medical – 30 degree head up bed rest, pneumovax vaccine, lactulose and avoid straining, antibiotics
- Surgical (ENT and neurosurgeons) – lumbar drain, repair of CSF fistula

Facial nerve palsy

- Consider high dose oral corticosteroids (1 mg/kg prednisolone, maximum 60 mg for 7 days then taper by 10 mg a day) while an inpatient
- Eye patch, lacrilube, viscotears, ophthalmology review

Hearing loss

- Consider high dose oral corticosteroids (1 mg/kg prednisolone, maximum 60 mg for 7 days then taper by 10 mg a day) depending on pattern and severity of hearing loss
- Outpatient considerations
  - Hearing aid
  - Follow-up with otology/audiology for counselling and consideration of hearing rehabilitation options, such as behind the ear (BTE) hearing aid, contralateral routing of sound (CROS) hearing aid, bone conducting hearing implant (BCHI) or ossicular chain reconstruction depending on cause, severity and pattern of hearing loss

Discharge and follow-up

- Discharge from hospital once all trauma-related injuries have been assessed.
- Follow-up depending on type of injuries.
  - Facial nerve palsy: Otology clinic for discussion of options – physiotherapy or surgical intervention, such as facial nerve decompression or repair.
  - Hearing loss: Otology/audiology clinic for consideration of hearing rehabilitation options.
  - Vertigo: Otology/balance clinic for Epley manoeuvre/vestibular rehabilitation.

RED FLAGS

- High-impact trauma
- Signs and symptoms of hearing loss, facial nerve palsy, CSF leak
- Other trauma-related injuries
- Reduced GCS/other neurological signs can represent intracranial pathology

Chapter 5

External ear trauma

Background

The external ear (pinna) is a cosmetically sensitive area and commonly subject to trauma by blunt or sharp injuries. A highly vascular area, the pinna consists of a cartilaginous framework covered on both sides by tightly adherent perichondrium and skin. Trauma to the pinna is classically due to lacerations, or blunt trauma, that can lead to the formation of a pinna haematoma. Both presentations need to be managed urgently to prevent long-term deformities. Pinna haematomas can have significant consequences if not managed promptly. The cartilage of the pinna receives its blood supply from the surrounding perichondrial layer and bleeding in the subperichondrial layer leads to formation of a haematoma. This rapidly results in avascular necrosis of the cartilage, deposition of fibronectin and a subsequent cauliflower ear deformity. Prompt recognition and management of such conditions can reduce the risk of such complications.

Potential areas for deterioration

D – risk of disability through neurosurgical sequelae of a high-impact trauma scenario

Preparation and equipment

- This is an ENT emergency, and the patient must be seen promptly.
- ENT may be asked to attend as a part of the formal trauma team in the event of polytrauma; a full ENT assessment is important in an ATLS approach:
  - The team should attend early to introduce themselves, assign roles and receive handover from the pre-hospital team if the patient is brought in by an ambulance.
  - Ensure the patient is assessed in accordance with the ATLS protocol with a primary survey.
  - Deal with any other potential injuries in order of priority according to trauma scenario.

History

Events

- Onset, timing and duration
- Laterality

DOI: 10.1201/b23238-7

- Preceding events
- Type of events – road traffic accident, assault, contact sport
- Post-event – loss of consciousness, blood loss, amnesia

Systems

- Ear – otalgia, otorrhoea (bloody, clear), tinnitus, vertigo, hearing loss, facial weakness
- Neurological (as part of a wider trauma screen) – headaches, syncope, seizures, loss of consciousness, vomiting

Red flags/risk factors

- High-impact trauma
- Hearing loss
- Facial nerve palsy
- CSF leak
- Severe vertigo
- Signs of pinna haematoma and overlying infection (abscess)

AMPLE

- Allergies, regular/recent medications, other relevant past medical history, time of last meal

Examination

- General inspection (ear) – lacerations, tissue loss, exposed cartilage, ecchymosis, fluctuant swelling
- General signs of temporal bone fracture – battle sign (postauricular ecchymosis), raccoon eyes (periorbital ecchymosis) (see temporal bone fracture chapter)
- Ear – palpation of swelling, otoscopy (bloody otorrhoea, CSF otorrhoea, hemotympanum, TM perforation)
- Neurological examination (if part of a wider trauma context)

Management

The principle of management in patients with ear trauma is dependent on the type and degree of trauma. The aim is to minimise cosmetic and functional impairment of the pinna and ear.

Pinna laceration (Figure 5.1)

- Assess and repair as soon as possible.
- Washout (saline/chlorhexidine/povidoiodine).
- Primary repair with direct closure to cover cartilage if no soft tissue loss (usually under local anaesthetic [LA]).
- Non-absorbable interrupted sutures are usually preferred (e.g. 4–0 or 5–0 prolene).
- Cartilage sutures are not necessarily required.
- In case of tissue loss, consider consulting local plastic surgery team.
- LA with adrenaline should be infiltrated as a pinna block and along the laceration site.
- Debride non-viable tissue.

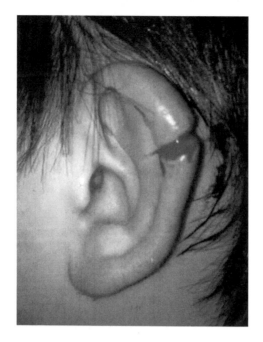

Figure 5.1 Pinna laceration.

Discharge and follow-up

- Discharge from hospital once successfully repaired (assuming no other head injuries)
- Antibiotics (5–7 days) to prevent infection
- Topical chloramphenicol ointment

Pinna haematoma (Figure 5.2)

- Assess and drain within 24 hours to minimise chance of avascular necrosis and long-term deformity
- Small haematoma (<1 cm) – needle aspiration to decompress haematoma
- Larger haematoma – incision and drainage (usually under LA)
- Prevent reaccumulation with compression – suture dental rolls each side of haematoma/ear splint and head bandage
- Superadded infection and cellulitis – consider admission for IV antibiotics, formal incision and drainage of abscess

Discharge and follow-up

- Discharge from hospital once injury is successfully repaired (assuming no other head injuries):
  - Antibiotics (5–7 days) to prevent infection
- Follow-up is usually in emergency clinic for:
  - Suture removal in 7–10 days

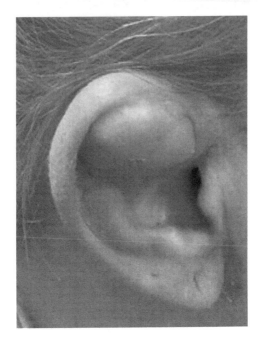

Figure 5.2 Pinna haematoma.

- Review of haematoma and recollection within 3–5 days
- Removal of head bandage and dental rolls within 3–5 days

WHEN TO REFER FROM PRIMARY CARE

To ED
- Suspected pinna haematoma/abscess

To emergency clinic
- Pinna cellulitis usually after antibiotic trial

Rhinology

Chapter 6

Epistaxis

Background

Epistaxis (nasal bleeding) is a common emergency that, in severe cases, has the potential for serious morbidity and mortality. Minor epistaxis episodes usually settle with simple first aid measures and such patients typically do not self-present to healthcare settings. Most cases of epistaxis are spontaneous in nature or preceded by trauma. Other, rarer, causes include clotting disorders, chronic granulomatous disorders or malignancy (such as angiofibroma, inverted papilloma or SCC). Risk factors for epistaxis include co-existing hypertension and the use of anticoagulant/antiplatelet medication. Although epistaxis can occur at any age, there is a bimodal distribution of cases with peaks in childhood and between 60 and 80 years. Most cases of epistaxis are anterior due to the rich vascular supply to the anterior nasal septum where Kiesselbach's plexus forms (also known as Little's area). Woodruff's plexus is found posterior to the inferior turbinate on the lateral nasal wall and is usually the area of bleeding found in the less common posterior epistaxis. The blood supply to the nasal cavity is derived from branches of the external and internal carotid arteries (Figure 6.1).

Potential areas of deterioration

A, B – risk of aspiration of blood causing airway obstruction or aspiration pneumonia – protect the airway by having the patient sit forward and spit out any blood in oropharynx

C – risk of hypovolaemic shock if blood loss is torrential and uncontrolled

Preparation and equipment

- This is an ENT emergency and assessment of the patient should be prioritised.
- Ask the ED team to apply direct pressure over the soft cartilaginous part of the nose, sit the patient upright and tilted forward.
- Attend with a headlight, nasal cautery equipment and nasal packs (anterior and posterior).

History

Symptoms

- Laterality (which side bled first)
- Time of onset, continuous or intermittent (estimated blood loss)

DOI: 10.1201/b23238-9

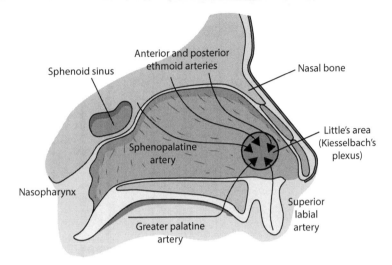

Figure 6.1 Schematic of the blood supply to the nasal septum. The anterior and posterior ethmoidal arteries are branches of the ophthalmic artery (branch of internal carotid). The sphenopalatine and greater palatine are branches of the maxillary artery (branch of the external carotid). The superior labial artery is a branch of the facial artery (branch of the external carotid).

- Measures employed to stop bleeding
- Preceding factors (e.g. trauma, anticoagulation)
- Previous episodes (especially requiring hospital admission)

Systems

- Nose – other discharge, anosmia, nasal obstruction, facial paraesthesia/anaesthesia/pain
- Hypovolaemia – pre-syncope/syncope, loss of consciousness, other bleeding

Risk factors/red flags

- Hypertension
- Clotting disorders
- Previous nasal surgery
- Anticoagulation or antiplatelet agents

AMPLE

- Allergies, regular/recent medications, other relevant past medical history, time of last meal

Examination

- Nose – anterior rhinoscopy to assess for anterior bleeding point or masses.
- Oropharynx – active bleeding in oropharynx can suggest posterior bleed.

- Full set of observations – assess for signs of hypovolaemia (tachycardia, hypotension, tachypnoea).

Management

The principle of management in patients with epistaxis is prompt haemorrhage control. This is a stepwise algorithm and can be achieved with simple first aid measures, cautery or nasal packing. Medical adjuncts can also be employed. Uncontrolled or persistent bleeding may require surgical intervention.

Simple first aid measures

- Pinch the soft cartilaginous part of the nose for 10–15 minutes and reassess.
- If no further bleeding, the patient can be observed for a short time and then discharged.

Cautery

- Anterior rhinoscopy to assess for a bleeding point (active bleeding/prominent vessel/clot) that can be a candidate for cautery.
- Silver nitrate 75% cautery stick +/− prior application of local anaesthetic.
- Gently roll cautery stick(s) around and then directly over bleeding point for 5–10 seconds (Figure 6.2).

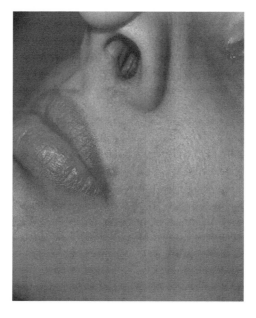

Figure 6.2 Post-nasal cautery with silver nitrate over a prominent blood vessel in Little's area of the nasal septum.

- Avoid cauterising both sides of the nasal septum in the same session (risk of septal necrosis/perforation).

Anterior packing

- Insert an 8–10-cm nasal pack (e.g. RapidRhino or Merocel) along the floor of the nose so the proximal end is flush with the nasal aperture (Figure 6.3).
- If using RapidRhino, soak the pack in sterile water for 30 seconds before insertion. Once in situ, inflate the balloon with air until the pilot cuff becomes rounded and feels firm when squeezed (10–12 mL).
- Pack contralateral side if bilateral epistaxis.
- Can use antero-posterior packs (if available) if bleeding remains uncontrolled.
- Analgesia and oral antibiotics if packs in situ >48 hours.

Posterior packing

- Foley catheter (male, 14 Fr) inserted along the floor of the nose to the nasopharynx
- Inflate with saline and pull back so the balloon is obstructing the choana
- Place umbilical clamp on catheter at the nasal aperture to maintain tension; apply gauze between clamp and skin to prevent alar necrosis
- Pack anterior nasal cavity with layered BIPP gauze or anterior pack

Medical adjuncts

- IV access with wide bore cannula.
- If the patient is being admitted, arrange full set of blood tests (especially FBC, clotting profile and group and save/crossmatch).
- Consider tranexamic acid (IV or oral).
- Reverse raised INR – vitamin K/beriplex – only after discussion with haematology team.

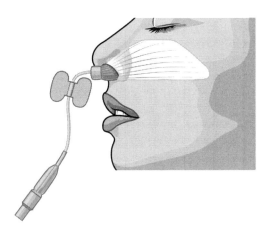

Figure 6.3 Anterior nasal pack properly sited on the floor of the nose flush with the entrance to the nasal passageway. Once inflated, it will occupy the majority of the nasal cavity to help stop the bleeding via a tamponade effect.

- Consider pausing anticoagulants/antiplatelets.
- Control elevated blood pressure.
- Ensure haemoglobin is stable and transfuse packed red cells if required.

Other methods

- Topical adrenaline-soaked cotton swabs can be placed in the nose when pinching or prior to cautery
- Haemostatic agents such as Floseal/Surgicel may be used if available
- Absorbable nasal packs such as Nasopore can be utilised but provide limited local pressure

Surgical

- Keep the patient nil by mouth (NBM).
- Consent the patient by explaining benefits, risks and alternatives.
- Surgical options include:
  - EUA and cautery (bipolar/monopolar diathermy, KTP LASER)
  - Endoscopic ligation of sphenopalatine artery (SPA)
  - Ligation of internal maxillary artery (Caldwell-Luc approach)
  - Open ligation of anterior ethmoidal artery (Lynch-Howarth incision)
  - Open ligation of external carotid artery
  - Interventional radiology – embolisation or coiling of feeding vessels

Discharge and follow-up

- If packed, patient is typically admitted with packs normally remaining in situ for 24 hours (often longer if coagulopathy).
- Once nasal packs are removed, identify any bleeding points for cautery.
- Discharge the patient with Naseptin cream (chlorhexidine gluconate, neomycin sulfate and peanut oil), Bactroban ointment (mupirocin) or Vaseline to anterior septum (to prevent nasal crusting and promote nasal mucosal health).
- If atypical presentation, patients may be followed-up in 4–6 weeks for full assessment of the nasal cavity to ensure there are no secondary causes of epistaxis such as malignancy.
- Safety net advice should be given on discharge regarding steps to take if rebleeding occurs.

RED FLAGS

- Patients with persistent uncontrollable epistaxis despite packing can deteriorate quickly and require urgent surgical intervention
- Active bleeding into the oropharynx despite anterior packing can represent a posterior bleed
- Deranged blood tests such as very high INR or low haemoglobin require medical optimisation
- Abnormal signs on examination such as nasal masses or repeated admissions for epistaxis can raise suspicions for a secondary cause such as malignancy

WHEN TO REFER FROM PRIMARY CARE

To ED
- Active bleeding that is unable to be controlled by simple first aid measures

To emergency clinic
- Regular presentations with spontaneous epistaxis for further assessment and cautery

To rhinology clinic via cancer referral pathway
- Suspicions of sinonasal malignancy (unilateral nasal obstruction and bloody discharge, facial pain, facial paraesthesia/anaesthesia) on a background of repeated epistaxis

Chapter 7

Orbital haematoma

Background

Orbital haematoma (or retrobulbar haemorrhage) is a rare but sight-threatening complication of endoscopic nasal surgery. It can also follow trauma and, very rarely, occur spontaneously. Trauma to branches of the ophthalmic artery (anterior and posterior ethmoidal arteries) or orbital vein can occur during common ENT procedures such as FESS or other endoscopic rhinological procedures. Damage to the vessel leads to blood accumulating in the confined space of the orbit, behind the globe. This results in an increase in intraorbital pressure, proptosis and, if untreated, visual loss.

Potential areas for deterioration

D – sight-threatening condition

Preparation and equipment

- This is an ENT and ophthalmological emergency, and the patient must be seen immediately.
- It is a sight-threatening, time-critical condition.
- Attend with or ask the theatre team to bring local anaesthetic, syringe with 27-gauge needle, iris scissors and artery clip.

History

Symptoms

- Onset, timing and duration
- Laterality
- Better or worse
- Operative details – what procedure, which side, indication, any perioperative complications, any abnormal anatomy

Systems

- Visual – change in vision, pain on eye movement, photophobia, blurred vision, retro-orbital pain
- Nose – epistaxis, CSF discharge (watery rhinorrhoea)
- Intracranial – nausea, vomiting, headache, loss of consciousness, seizures

DOI: 10.1201/b23238-10

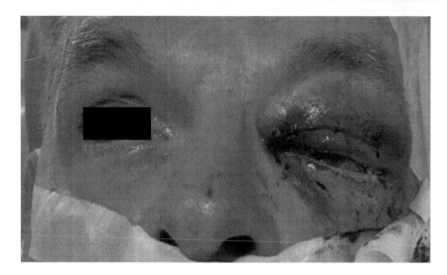

Figure 7.1 Clinical image of a patient with a left-sided orbital haematoma following endoscopic rhinological surgery.

AMPLE

- Allergies, regular/recent medications, other relevant past medical history, time of last meal

Examination

- Eye – general inspection, lid oedema, ecchymosis, ability to open, subconjunctival haemorrhage, proptosis/chemosis (Figure 7.1)
- Vision – current vision compared to baseline (no change, blurring, colour, shadow, movement)
- Cranial nerves:
  - II (optic) – fields, acuity, relative afferent pupillary defect (RAPD), colour, pupillary reflexes
  - III (oculomotor), IV (trochlear), VI (abducens) – diplopia, ophthalmoplegia, eye movement
- Nose – anterior rhinoscopy to assess for epistaxis or CSF rhinorrhoea
- Full set of observations

Management

The principle of management in patients with orbital haematoma is urgent recognition and decompression of the orbit to prevent visual loss. Ideally, this is done with a return to the operation theatre but often will require a bedside canthotomy and cantholysis for urgent decompression to buy time to return to the theatre.

Immediate – lateral canthotomy/cantholysis (Figure 7.2)

- Urgent bedside measure to help buy time prior to formal orbital decompression.
- Removal of any nasal packs.

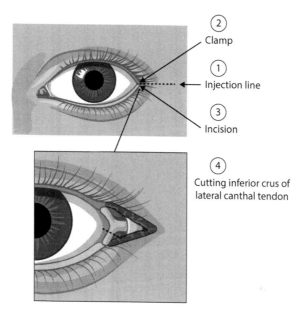

Figure 7.2 **Steps required to perform canthotomy and cantholysis to the lateral canthal tendon** of the eyelids.

- Infiltrate local anaesthetic (2% lidocaine and 1:80,000 adrenaline) to lateral canthus.
- Apply artery clip for 1 minute to reduce blood supply to the bony orbit.
- Sharp straight iris scissors to the lateral canthal angle (canthotomy).
- Rotate scissors 90 degrees to cut through lateral canthal tendon (cantholysis).
- Cut deep to the skin through the orbital septum and conjunctiva below the tarsal plate to allow drainage of the haematoma.
- A tonometer can be used to measure the intraocular pressure (<20 mmHg is normal).

Medical – reduce intraorbital pressure with medication

- 1 g/kg IV mannitol over 30 minutes
- 500 mg IV acetazolamide
- 0.5% topical timolol

Surgical – proceed to endoscopic orbital decompression as the definitive treatment if concerns about vision

- Removal of laminal papyracea.
- Dissection to locate the bleeding vessel is not usually required as this can cause further damage and vasospasm of the culprit vessel usually ensues.

Discharge and follow-up

- Admit the patient for observation and monitoring for signs of further bleeding/ visual compromise.

- Urgent inpatient ophthalmology review.
- Outpatient follow-up with ENT and ophthalmology teams.

RED FLAGS

- Rapid onset swelling
- Tense orbit shortly after sinus surgery
- Loss of colour vision (early sign)

Chapter 8

Periorbital cellulitis

Background

Periorbital cellulitis is a potentially sight-threatening condition. While the inflammatory origins in preseptal periorbital cellulitis derive from the skin of the eyelid, postseptal cellulitis is a complication of acute rhinosinusitis (ARS), with infection spreading from the paranasal sinuses to the orbit. Most commonly seen in children, orbital complications of ARS are associated with bacterial infection of the ethmoid and maxillary sinuses, and less commonly frontal and sphenoid sinuses. Typical causative organisms are *Haemophilus influenzae, Streptococcus pneumonia* or *Staphylococcus spp.* Table 8.1 highlights the Chandler classification which shows the different stages of periorbital cellulitis.

Potential areas of deterioration

C – risk of developing septic shock
D – sight-threatening condition and intracranial extension of infection

Preparation and equipment

- This is an ENT emergency, and the patient must be seen promptly.
- Involve members of the MDT early, including paediatricians and ophthalmologists.

History

Symptoms

- Onset, timing and duration
- Laterality
- Better or worse
- Preceding symptoms of rhinosinusitis (anosmia, rhinorrhoea, nasal congestion, facial pain) or coryza
- Previous episodes including previous hospital admissions and previous treatments and their effects

Systems

- Visual – change in vision/colour vision, pain on eye movement, retro-orbital pain, photophobia

DOI: 10.1201/b23238-11

Table 8.1 Chandler classification of periorbital cellulitis

Stage	Type	Description
Stage I	Preseptal cellulitis	Infection of tissues anterior to the orbital septum
Stage II	Orbital cellulitis	Infection of the orbit
Stage III	Subperiosteal abscess	Abscess formation between the periorbita and sinuses
Stage IV	Orbital abscess	Abscess formation within the space defined by the ocular muscles (intraconal)
Stage V	Cavernous sinus thrombosis	Spread of infection to the veins and cavernous sinus

- Intracranial – nausea, vomiting, headache, loss of consciousness, seizures, rashes, features of meningism

Risk factors/red flags

- States of immunocompromise
- Rapid deterioration
- Signs of cavernous sinus thrombosis – severe headache with retro-orbital pain, bulging eye, double vision, fever, reduced visual acuity, bilateral eye signs, involvement of cranial nerves III, IV, V1/V2 and VI, evolving neurological signs and reduced GCS

AMPLE

- Allergies, regular/recent medications, other relevant past medical history, time of last meal
- Paediatrics – antenatal and obstetric complications, developmental history and immunisation status

Examination

- Eye – general inspection, lid oedema, ecchymosis, ability to open, subconjunctival haemorrhage, proptosis/chemosis
- Vision – current vision compared to baseline (no change, blurring, colour, shadow, movement)
- Cranial nerves:
  - II (optic) – fields, acuity, RAPD, colour vision, pupillary reflexes
  - III (oculomotor), IV (trochlear), VI (abducens) – diplopia, ophthalmoplegia, eye movement
  - V1 (ophthalmic branch of trigeminal), V2 (maxillary branch of trigeminal) – impaired corneal reflex and sensation to facial skin
- Nose – assess for signs of rhinosinusitis with anterior rhinoscopy or flexible nasoendoscopy (FNE) (pus at middle meatus, oedema, erythema, congestion)
- Neurological – GCS, assess for signs of meningism (nuchal rigidity, non-blanching rash, Kernig's sign, Brudzinski's sign)
- Full set of observations – assess for signs of sepsis (fever, tachycardia, hypotension, tachypnoea)

Management

The principle in management for patients with periorbital cellulitis is to treat the infection with antimicrobials/drainage and decongest the nose to allow the sinuses to drain. This is usually achieved medically but may escalate to surgery if there is a subperiosteal/orbital abscess or intracranial extension. Workup with swabs, bloods and imaging are useful adjuncts to help guide management.

Bedside investigations

- Swab – eye swab and nasal swab sent for mc&s
- Bloods – FBC, U&Es, CRP, blood cultures, VBG with lactate

Imaging

- Contrast CT scan of orbit and brain indicated in (Figure 8.1):
  - Paediatric patients
  - Patients not responding to IV antibiotics
  - Unable to examine the eye
  - Suspicions of abscess (proptosis, ophthalmoplegia, reduced visual acuity) or cavernous sinus thrombosis (bilateral eye signs with neurology)
- MRI brain with contrast – intracranial extension

Medical

- Antibiotics to cover aerobic and anaerobic bacteria.
  - IV is the usual route of choice; oral antibiotics may be suitable in uncomplicated preseptal cellulitis.

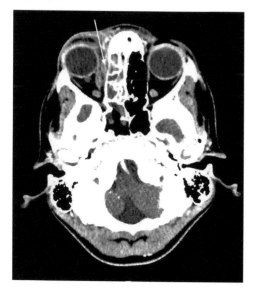

Figure 8.1 Axial CT head and orbits showing right-sided orbital and periorbital cellulitis with subperiosteal abscess/collection overlying the right lamina papyracea (white arrow). There is associated right-sided paranasal sinus mucosal thickening involving the right ethmoid sinus.

- Convert to oral antibiotics once afebrile for 48 hours and evidence of resolving signs and symptoms.
- IV fluids (20 mL/kg as initial paediatric resuscitation).
- Nasal decongestant – facilitate sinus drainage.
- Topical (intranasal) corticosteroids and nasal douching to manage acute rhinosinusitis (ARS).
- Analgesia.

Surgical

- Keep the patient NBM.
- Informed consent of the patient by explaining benefits, risks and alternatives
- Surgical intervention is indicated when radiological evidence of an abscess, failure to respond to IV antibiotic therapy after 24–48 hours and if concerns regarding intracranial extension.
- Surgical drainage of abscess with either:
  - Open (Lynch Howarth incision) to medial, superior and superolateal abscesses (Figure 8.2).
  - Endoscopic approach – open lamina papyracea and ethmoidectomy.
- Sinus washout with functional endoscopic sinus surgery (FESS).
- Intracranial extension requires neurosurgical input.
- Post-operatively continue antibiotics, review mc&s results and adjust antibiotic therapy accordingly.
- Regular ENT and ophthalmology reviews.

Cavernous sinus thrombosis

- IV antibiotics, IV fluids, IV corticosteroids
- Surgical drainage (usually sphenoid sinus)
- Anticoagulants – debated but commonly used if no contraindications

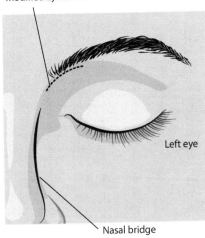

Figure 8.2 Location of a Lynch-Howarth curvilinear incision in relation to the nasal bridge, medial brow and eye.

Discharge and follow-up

- Patients can be considered for discharged once they have been converted to oral antibiotics.
- Discharged patients to complete a course of oral antibiotics and to continue with treatment of rhinosinusitis.
- Follow-up decided between paediatrics, ENT and ophthalmology teams – may involve a combination of multiple specialties.

RED FLAGS

- Inability to open and examine the eye
- Signs and symptoms of abscess – severe headache with retro-orbital pain, bulging eye, double vision, fever, reduced visual acuity
- Signs and symptoms of cavernous sinus thrombosis – bilateral eye signs, neurological signs, such as reduced GCS
- Failure to respond to IV antibiotics within 24–48 hours
- Signs of abscess or intracranial extension on imaging

WHEN TO REFER FROM PRIMARY CARE

To ED

- Sick, toxic-looking child/patient
- Failure to respond to oral antibiotics
- Unable to open and examine the eye
- Signs of shock with tachycardia, high pyrexia and low blood pressure
- Signs and symptoms of orbital abscess or cavernous sinus thrombosis

Chapter 9

Nasal trauma

Background

Nasal trauma is common in all ages and can have a range of complicating injuries. The external nasal anatomy can be divided into thirds. The upper third consists of the paired nasal bones which meet the frontal bone at the nasion. Laterally, the nasal bones articulate with the frontal process of the maxilla. These form a pyramidal shape at the bridge of the nose. The middle and lower thirds are made of the upper and lower lateral cartilages. The anatomical cartilaginous and bony structures of the nose are shown in Figure 9.1. Broadly speaking, sensory innervation is via the trigeminal nerve (ophthalmic and maxillary divisions), blood supply is from both the internal and external carotid arteries and venous drainage is via the facial vein and valveless pharyngeal and pterygoid plexuses. This chapter will discuss nasal fractures and septal haematomas. Nasal bone fractures should be identified, assessed and, if necessary, manipulated early before callous formation, approximately 2–3 weeks after injury. Septal haematomas are a result of blood accumulating in the mucoperichondrium. These should be drained immediately to prevent subsequent septal abscess or ischaemic necrosis of the septum and resulting saddle nose deformity. Septal abscesses can lead to intracranial sepsis due to infection spreading through the valveless venous system draining the nose.

Potential areas for deterioration

D – risk of intracranial sepsis from a septal abscess

Preparation and equipment

- Attend the patient with Thudicum's speculum and a headlight.
- ENT may be asked to attend as part of the formal trauma team in the event of polytrauma; a full ENT assessment is important in an ATLS approach:
  - The team should attend early to introduce themselves, assign roles and receive handover from the pre-hospital team if the patient is brought in by an ambulance.
  - Ensure the patient is assessed in accordance with the ATLS protocol with a primary survey.
  - Deal with any other potential injuries in order of priority according to trauma scenario.

DOI: 10.1201/b23238-12

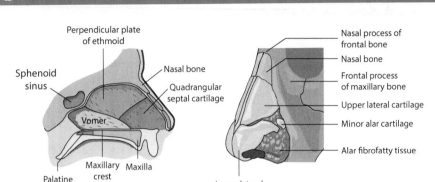

Figure 9.1 Cartilaginous and bony anatomy of the nose.

History

Events

- Preceding events
- Type of events – road traffic accident, assault, contact sport
- Post-event – loss of consciousness, blood loss, amnesia

Systems

- Nose – epistaxis, other nasal discharge, change in appearance, nasal airway obstruction, facial pain
- Intracranial – nausea, vomiting, headache, loss of consciousness, seizures, rashes, features of meningism

Red flags/risk factors

- High-impact trauma
- Septal haematoma
- Signs and symptoms of septal necrosis or intracranial infection

AMPLE

- Allergies, regular/recent medications, other relevant past medical history, time of last meal

Examination

- General signs of nasal bone fracture – periorbital bruising, clear deviation, significant swelling around nasal bridge
- Nose – change in appearance, lacerations, facial paraesthesia, bite malalignment
- Septal haematoma – bilateral, boggy (deviated septal cartilage is unilateral and hard)
- Full set of observations

Management

The principle of management in patients with nasal trauma is to identify the nasal injuries and manage these accordingly. Nasal bone fractures are usually managed in emergency clinics 5–7 days after injury, as facial swelling often obscures examination findings and the ability to assess for a true deviation. Septal haematomas should be drained on a more urgent basis, usually under general anaesthesia.

Imaging

- Routine imaging is not indicated in isolated nasal trauma
- CT head with contrast is indicated if there are concerns regarding intracranial extension from a septal abscess

Nasal bone fracture

- Can be managed conservatively or surgically (manipulation under anaesthesia, manipulation under anaesthesia [MUA]).
- MUA is indicated to straighten a newly laterally deviated nose.
  - Between 10 and 21 days of injury.
  - Local anaesthetic infiltration to infratrochlear and external branch of anterior ethmoidal nerves.
  - Manipulate the nasal bones first caudally (towards the chin) then back towards the midline.
  - Paediatric patients and more complicated cases can be manipulated under general anaesthetic.

Septal haematoma

- Confirm presence via aspiration of blood with a needle and syringe under local anaesthetic spray
- Definitive drainage within 24 hours to reduce risk of septal necrosis
  - Incision and drainage is preferred over needle aspiration which has a high reaccumulation rate
  - Through-and-through absorbable sutures placed into the septum and nasal packs to reduce risk of reaccumulation
  - More complicated cases may require placement of corrugated drains and bilateral nasal packs

Septal abscess

- Definitive drainage under general anaesthetic as described above
- Swabs pus and send for mc&s
- Admit under ENT for IV antibiotics and monitoring for intracranial extension

Discharge and follow-up

- Patients undergoing an MUA under local or general anaesthetic can be discharged on the same day and advised to avoid contact sports for 6–8 weeks.
- Patients with septal haematoma can be discharged after 24–48 hours if no evidence of reaccumulation.
- Patients with septal abscess can be discharged to complete a course of oral antibiotics once there are clinical signs that they are improving on IV antibiotics.
- Nasal packs following incision and drainage can be removed after 24–48 hours.
- Any residual nasal deformity after MUA or persistent nasal obstruction symptoms may require further surgery. This should be delayed until at least 6 months

post-injury to allow bony remodelling to occur. Consult with a rhinologist for consideration of septoplasty/septorhinoplasty.

- Follow-up patients with a drainage septal haematoma/abscess in rhinology clinic to assess for any complications/nasal deformities.

RED FLAGS

- Septal haematoma/abscess
- Signs and symptoms of intracranial extension

WHEN TO REFER FROM PRIMARY CARE

To ED

- Suspected septal haematoma/abscess

To emergency clinic (5–7 days post-injury)

- Isolated suspected nasal bone fracture

Head and neck

Chapter 10

Adult acute airway obstruction

Background

Adults with acute airway obstruction can present with noisy breathing, respiratory distress or unresponsiveness/respiratory arrest. It carries a high mortality rate, and many patients will not survive to hospital. Noisy breathing can be a sign of upper or lower respiratory obstruction, and it is important to distinguish each of these to ensure the patient is managed by the correct medical team (ENT or respiratory medicine). Stridor is a harsh, high-pitched, added airway sound that suggests obstructed soft tissue in the larynx or upper trachea. It is usually inspiratory but also can be expiratory and lower pitched if the obstruction is more distal in the subglottis and thoracic trachea. Biphasic stridor usually represents a more severe obstruction. Stertor is a low, vibratory upper airway sound similar to snoring that suggests obstruction at the level of the oropharynx. Wheeze is a high-pitched whistling sound that is usually expiratory and represents soft tissue obstruction of the intrathoracic airway and lungs. There are many different causes of airway obstruction in adults (Table 10.1), from new acute conditions (such as epiglottitis/supraglottitis) to acute on chronic presentations (progression of laryngeal malignancy). If a patient presents with life-threatening airway compromise, this should be immediately managed and the airway secured, taking precedence over taking a history, thorough examination and investigations.

Potential areas of deterioration

A – risk of airway obstruction progressing to respiratory arrest and death

Preparation and equipment

- This is a critical ENT emergency, and the patient should be assessed immediately.
- Ensure the patient is in an appropriate high-dependency area with the difficult airway equipment available.
- Call the anaesthetic team to attend alongside you.
- Bring headlight, tongue depressor and fibreoptic nasendoscope.
- Make senior colleague aware that you have a potential airway concern.

Immediate assessment

- Perform a rapid A to E assessment before proceeding either with immediate resuscitation or taking a history from patient/relative/ambulance crew
- If the patient presents in cardiorespiratory arrest, then commence CPR and resuscitation according to ALS guidelines with the appropriate teams notified

DOI: 10.1201/b23238-14

Table 10.1 Causes of acute upper airway obstruction in adults

Structural	Foreign body, bilateral vocal cord palsy, subglottic stenosis
Infection	Epiglottitis, supraglottitis, Ludwig's angina, deep space neck infections
Inflammation	Anaphylaxis, angioedema, autoimmune (SLE, rheumatoid arthritis, systemic sclerosis, granulomatosis with polyangiitis)
Malignancy	Tongue base, laryngeal, thyroid (and goitre), oesophageal, mediastinal, papillomatosis
Trauma	Penetrating or blunt, laryngeal fracture, airway burn
Iatrogenic	Bilateral recurrent laryngeal nerve surgical injury, post thyroidectomy haematoma

History

Symptoms

- Onset, timing and duration
- Intermittent/continuous
- Exacerbating or relieving factors
- Previous episodes (especially requiring admission to hospital/ICU)
- Trauma history
- Known history of head and neck malignancy

Systems

- Airway – SOB, aspiration/choking, drooling
- Oesophagus – rapid onset dysphagia, odynophagia, regurgitation
- Voice – rapid onset of change in voice

Risk factors/red flags

- Referred otalgia, hoarse voice, neck lump, haemoptysis, weight loss
- Smoking, alcohol
- Family history of laryngeal malignancy

AMPLE

- Allergies, regular/recent medications, other relevant past medical history, time of last meal

Examination

- General inspection for signs of respiratory distress – noisy breathing (stridor, stertor), tachypnoea, cyanosis, use of accessory muscles, anxiety, agitation, fatigue
- Voice – speaking in full sentences, quality of voice, hoarseness
- Neck – range of motion and torticollis, lumps, cellulitis
- Oral cavity/oropharynx – tongue and floor of mouth swelling, tonsils, peritonsillar swelling
- Flexible nasoendoscopy (FNE) – mucous membrane swelling, generalised oedema, pharyngeal asymmetry, supraglottitis, epiglottitis, foreign body, vocal cord movement, laryngeal mass, subglottic stenosis

- Chest – palpation for surgical emphysema and auscultation for signs of aspiration
- Full set of observations – assess for signs of respiratory distress (tachypnoea, reduced saturations) or sepsis (tachycardia, fever, hypotension)

Management

The principle of management in adults with acute airway obstruction is to maintain effective gas exchange via a safe airway. This may require securing a definitive airway (endotracheal intubation or front of neck access) or medical management strategies that can be employed in less critical presentations. The order in which you perform your history, examination and management should adapt to the situation in front of you, which may be rapidly evolving. Management of such patients typically requires an MDT approach with senior ENT, anaesthetic/critical care, and ED colleagues on hand.

Bedside

- Sit patient up.
- Monitor saturations and oxygenate (15 L high-flow oxygen or high-flow nasal cannula [HFNC] therapy).
- Heliox can buy time if immediately available (21% oxygen, 79% helium) – has a lower density than air which improves oxygen delivery to the airways.
- IV corticosteroids.
- Nebulisers – adrenaline and/or corticosteroids.
- Specific immediate bedside management depending on underlying cause (e.g. IM adrenaline for anaphylaxis).
- Bloods – specific to underlying cause (e.g. FBC, U&E, CRP, lactate, blood cultures, autoimmune screen)

Imaging

- Consider CT neck/thorax with contrast – assess for any structural abnormality of the upper airways

Conservative/medical

- Admit the patient for close observations.
- Continue with IV corticosteroid, nebulisers, oxygen, heliox as indicated.
- Consider specific treatment depending on the cause (e.g. IV antibiotics for epiglottitis).
- Discuss options for further management and next steps with the patient when he/she is stable.
- Make critical care teams aware that if the patient is not being admitted to ICU/HDU and have a plan for steps to be taken if the condition of the patient deteriorates.

Surgical – secure a definitive airway (endotracheal tube or front of neck access)

- Keep the patient NBM.
- If able, get informed consent of the patient by explaining benefits, risks and alternatives.
- ENT surgical team scrubbed with difficult airway trolley and tracheostomy kit in case of failed intubation.
- In cases of epiglottis, consider an epiglottic swab for mc&s during intubation.

- Work closely with the anaesthetist and have a clear plan prior to the procedure; this could be:
  - Facemask ventilation and endotracheal intubation (at end of direct laryngoscopy, video laryngoscopy, bougie or fibreoptic nasal intubation (maximum 3+1 attempts).
- Emergency front of neck access (FONA) should only be performed in "can't intubate, can't ventilate scenario":
  - Surgical tracheostomy – preferred, safer, longer procedure.
  - Scalpel cricothyroidotomy (Figure 10.1).
    - Transverse stab incision through cricothyroid membrane with 10 blade.
    - Turn blade 90 degrees to move the sharp edge caudally.
    - Insert bougie into trachea along the blade.
    - Railroad lubricated 6 mm cuffed endotracheal tube into trachea.
    - Confirm the position and secure the tube.
- Transfer the patient to ICU for post-operative care and close monitoring.
- Patients should continue their medical therapy following placement of a secure airway as appropriate – for example, IV antibiotics to treat epiglottitis.
- The decision to extubate/decannulate should be made with an MDT approach.
  - Irreversible/progressive cause of airway obstruction require a long-term tracheostomy.

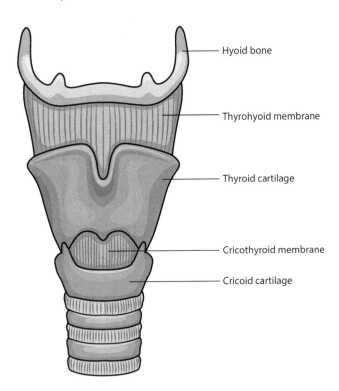

Figure 10.1 **Anatomical schematic of the larynx. Emergency surgical cricothyroidotomy** should be performed at the cricothyroid membrane.

Chapter 11

Acute paediatric airway obstruction

Background

Paediatric acute airway obstruction tends to have different causes and management compared to adults. Clinical presentation can vary from noisy breathing to complete obstruction and respiratory arrest; it, therefore, carries a high potential for mortality. Added airway sounds include stridor, stertor or wheeze (described in the acute adult airway obstruction chapter). There are a wide variety of potential aetiologies (Table 11.1), including congenital causes and upper airway infections. A normally healthy child can tolerate some degree of airway obstruction, maintaining tidal volume close to the point of exhaustion. After this, there is a rapid decompensation with hypoxaemia, hypercapnia, acidosis and, ultimately, respiratory arrest. Clinical parameters, such as tachypnoea, increased respiratory effort, reduced air entry, cyanosis and reduced consciousness, are good measures to predict respiratory failure. Like adults, if patients present with any immediate life-threatening airway concerns, this should be managed and secured appropriately before assessing for a cause.

Potential areas of deterioration

A – risk of airway obstruction progressing to respiratory arrest and death

Preparation and equipment

- This is an ENT emergency, and the patient should be seen immediately.
- Ensure the patient is in paediatric resus with the difficult airway trolley available.
- Call the anaesthetic and paediatric teams to attend alongside you.
- Make senior colleague aware that you have a potential airway concern.

Immediate assessment

- Perform a rapid A to E assessment before proceeding either with immediate resuscitation or taking a history from parent/ambulance crew.
- If the patient presents in cardiorespiratory arrest, then commence CPR and resuscitation according to paediatric BLS guidelines with the appropriate teams notified.

DOI: 10.1201/b23238-15

Table 11.1 Causes of acute paediatric airway obstruction

Structural	Foreign body, bilateral vocal cord palsy, laryngomalacia, laryngeal web, subglottic haemangioma
Infection	Croup, epiglottitis, supraglottitis, bacterial tracheitis, deep neck space infection
Inflammation	Anaphylaxis, angioedema
Trauma	Penetrating or blunt
Iatrogenic	Bilateral recurrent laryngeal nerve surgical injury, tracheal/ laryngeal injury
Congenital	Micrognathia, choanal atresia, subglottic stenosis, laryngeal atresia

History

Symptoms

- Onset, timing and duration
- Intermittent/continuous
- Exacerbating or relieving factors – especially crying, feeding or positional
- Associated symptoms – fever, drowsiness, loss of consciousness
- Previous episodes (especially requiring admission to hospital/NICU/PICU)

Systems

- Airway – SOB, aspiration/choking, drooling
- Oesophagus – rapid onset dysphagia, odynophagia, regurgitation
- Voice – rapid onset change in voice

Paediatric history

- Birth history – antenatal complications, gestational age at birth, mode of delivery/ complications
- Neonatal history – intubation, NICU stay, neonatal illnesses
- Developmental history – conditions associated with low muscle tone such as Down's syndrome, cerebral palsy, muscular dystrophy, immunisation history

AMPLE

- Allergies, regular/recent medications, other relevant past medical history, time of last meal

Examination

The main variance in managing paediatric compared to adult airway obstruction is to recognise children who are at risk of worsening their obstruction with examination. If a child is in distress, then you should avoid disturbing them. Allow them to remain as calm as possible by keeping them with their parent/guardian, performing as much of the examination away from them as possible. Examination of the oropharynx and chest should only be performed if the child is settled and allowing you to proceed with this examination. Paediatric FNE should only be performed once by a senior ENT doctor if the child is compliant and settled.

- General inspection for signs of respiratory distress – noisy breathing (stridor, stertor), tachypnoea, cyanosis, use of accessory muscles, tracheal tug, nasal flaring, agitation
- Signs of exhaustion – bradypnoea, reduced air entry, reduced respiratory effort, quiet stridor, decreased conscious level
- Craniofacial morphology – assess for signs of congenital abnormalities, syndromes, sequences and obvious structural abnormalities such as retro/micrognathia
- Voice – speaking in full sentences, quality of voice, hoarseness
- Neck – range of motion/torticollis, neck lumps, cellulitis
- Oral cavity/oropharynx – tongue and floor of mouth swelling, tonsils, peritonsillar swelling
- Chest – auscultation for signs of aspiration, reduced air entry
- Full set of observations – assess for signs of respiratory distress (tachypnoea, reduced saturations) or sepsis (tachycardia, fever, hypotension)

Management

The principle of management in paediatric patients with acute airway obstruction is to maintain a safe airway and prevent further deterioration. It is imperative that the child is not distressed during this process as this could worsen their condition. Allow them to remain calm. This may include allowing parents/guardians to apply face masks to deliver oxygen and other medications. Paediatricians, critical care and ED colleagues should be on hand and have an input into the shared management of these high-risk patients. The following are examples of management strategies that can be employed depending on the patient and the cause of their airway obstruction. It is important to be flexible with your history, examination, investigation and management steps so that you are able to adapt to the evolving situation in front of you. It may be necessary to first secure the airway with a definitive airway before performing invasive investigations, including cannulation.

Bedside

- Sit patient up.
- Monitor saturations and oxygenate (15 L high flow oxygen).
- Heliox can buy time if available (21% oxygen, 79% helium) – has a lower density than air which improves oxygen delivery to the airways.
- IV corticosteroids.
- Nebulisers – adrenaline or budesonide.
- Specific immediate bedside management depending on the cause (e.g. IM adrenaline for anaphylaxis).
- Bloods – specific to underlying cause (e.g. FBC, U&E, CRP, lactate, blood cultures, autoimmune screen).

Imaging

- Consider CT neck and thorax with contrast - assess for any structural abnormality of the upper airways

Conservative/medical

- Admit the patient for close observations.
- Continue with IV steroids, nebulisers, oxygen, heliox as indicated.
- Consider specific treatment depending on the cause (e.g. IV antibiotics for epiglottitis).
- Discuss options for further management and next steps with the parents when the patient is stable.

Surgical – definitive airway (endotracheal tube or tracheostomy)

- Keep the patient NBM.
- If able, get the informed consent of the parent/guardian by explaining benefits, risks and alternatives.
- ENT surgical team scrubbed with difficult airway trolley and tracheostomy kit in case of failed intubation.
- In cases of epiglottis, consider an epiglottic swab for mc&s during intubation.
- Work closely with the anaesthetist and have a clear plan prior to the procedure, this is usually:
  - Gas induction
  - Tracheal intubation either with direct laryngoscopy, video laryngoscopy, bougie or fibroptic nasoendoscopic intubation (maximum 3+1 attempts)
- Emergency front of neck access (FONA) should only be performed in "can't intubate, can't ventilate scenario":
  - Surgical tracheostomy – preferred, safer, longer procedure.
  - Scalpel cricothyroidotomy.
    - Transverse stab incision through cricothyroid membrane with 10 blade.
    - Turn blade 90 degrees to move the sharp edge caudally.
    - Insert bougie into trachea along the blade.
    - Railroad lubricated 6 mm cuffed endotracheal tube into the trachea.
    - Confirm the position and secure the tube.
- Once the airway is secure then the appropriate treatment can occur depending on the cause, for example:
  - Ventilating bronchoscopes and jet ventilation for retrieving airway foreign bodies.
  - IV antibiotics to treat epiglottitis.
- Transfer the patient to PICU for post-operative care and close monitoring.
  - This may require transfer to a specialist unit.
- The decision to extubate/decannulate should be made with an MDT approach.

Chapter 12

Penetrating and blunt neck trauma

Background

Trauma to the neck may be penetrating or blunt. Both carry with them a risk of mortality and damage to structures in the neck, including the upper aerodigestive tract, major vessels and nerves, cervical spine and spinal cord, thyroid and salivary glands. Penetrating neck injuries are more common than blunt injuries and can be due to stab wounds or high-velocity injuries (including incidents involving firearms). Blunt injuries can cause injury through high-impact force, most commonly following a road traffic accident, assault or neck ligation. The location of injury is categorised according to its anatomical zone (Table 12.1). This theoretically helps identify patients who may need surgical exploration alongside the hard and soft signs that can guide management. As with all trauma scenarios, it is important that these are managed in a systematic manner with the most life-threatening injuries addressed first.

Potential areas for deterioration

A – risk of airway compromise through contained haemorrhage causing compression or direct laryngo-tracheal injury

C – risk of major haemorrhage through direct injury of major neck vessels

D – risk of disability through nervous injury or compromised cerebral blood flow through transected internal carotid artery

Preparation and equipment

- This is an ENT emergency, and the patient must be seen immediately.
- ENT may be asked to attend as part of the formal trauma team in the event of polytrauma; a full ENT assessment is important in an ATLS approach:
  - The team should attend early to introduce themselves, assign roles and receive handover from the pre-hospital team if the patient is brought in by an ambulance.
  - Ensure the patient is assessed in accordance with the ATLS protocol with a primary survey.
  - Deal with any other potential injuries in order of priority according to trauma scenario.

DOI: 10.1201/b23238-16

Table 12.1 Anatomical zones of the neck for penetrating neck trauma and their contents

Zone	Boundaries	Contents at risk
1	Sternal notch to cricoid cartilage	Organs – trachea, oesophagus Vasculature – subclavian artery and vein, jugular and innominate veins, common carotid and vertebral arteries Nerves – vagus and recurrent laryngeal, brachial plexus, spinal cord
2	Cricoid cartilage to angle of mandible	Organs – larynx, pharynx, submandibular gland Vasculature – vertebral, common carotid, internal and external carotid arteries, jugular veins Nerves – vagus, spinal cord
3	Angle of mandible to skull base	Vasculature – internal carotid, external carotid and vertebral arteries, jugular veins Nerves – glossopharyngeal, vagus, spinal accessory, hypoglossal, spinal cord

History

Events

- Preceding events
- Type of events – road traffic accident, assault
- Post event – difficulty breathing, blood loss, amnesia

Systems

- Airway – SOB, aspiration/choking, drooling, coughing/haemoptysis
- Oesophagus – dysphagia, odynophagia, haematemesis
- Voice – change in voice
- Neurological – loss of consciousness, paraesthesia, paralysis

Red flags/risk factors

- High-impact trauma
- Active bleeding

AMPLE

- Allergies, regular/recent medications, other relevant past medical history, time of last meal

Examination

- General inspection – active bleeding, weapon in situ, patient's consciousness level
- Respiratory distress – noisy breathing (stridor, stertor), tachypnoea, cyanosis, use of accessory muscles, anxiety, agitation, fatigue
- Examine for hard and soft clinical features of penetrating neck injury from history and examination (Table 12.2)
- Neck – subcutaneous emphysema, reduced range of motion
  - Penetrating neck injury – expansile, pulsatile masses
  - Blunt neck injury – bruising, tenderness on palpation of larynx

Table 12.2 Hard and soft clinical features of penetrating neck injuries

	Hard clinical features	Soft clinical features
History	Haematemesis Airway compromise	Minor haematemesis Dysphagia Dyspnoea Paraesthesia
Examination	Expanding/pulsatile haematoma Active bleeding Airway compromise Shock Neurological deficit including paralysis	Expanding haematoma Subcutaneous emphysema Venous ooze

- Oral cavity – if suspicions of breach through floor of the mouth or palate
- Cranial nerves and neurological examination
- FNE – active bleeding, mucosal tears, laryngeal oedema, signs of laryngotracheal disruption and other causes of airway compromise such as vocal cord palsy
- Full set of observations – assess for signs of hypovolemic shock (tachycardia, hypotension)

Management

Following patient stabilisation, the principle of managing patients with neck trauma is to identify the extent of any injury and treat accordingly. These may range from superficial neck lacerations that can be managed with simple wound closure under local anaesthesia to life-changing injuries involving critical neck structures. If there are concerns regarding airway compromise, then immediate steps should be taken to secure a definitive airway (see chapter on acute adult airway obstruction).

Bedside investigations

- Blood tests – FBC, U&Es, coagulation profile, group and save/crossmatch as part of the trauma scenario

Imaging

- CT traumogram will likely be conducted as part of the trauma scenario
- CT head and neck with contrast/angiogram
  - Signs of vascular injury – transection, occlusion, active bleeding, pseudoaneurysm, dissection, arteriovenous fistula, intimal injury, perivascular haematoma/fat stranding/gas (Figure 12.1)
  - Signs of organ injury (larynx, trachea, oesophagus) – direct injury, air tracking, subcutaneous emphysema

General

- Consider tetanus booster and/or tranexamic acid
- Analgesia

Non-operative

- Close observations in monitored area for signs of deterioration
- Head up nursing to reduce impact of any laryngeal oedema

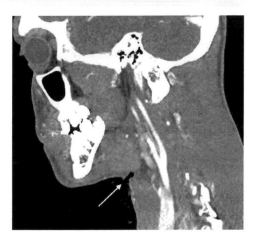

Figure 12.1 Sagittal CT head and neck showing a soft tissue wound tract is seen extending 1 cm medially just below the level of the right submandibular gland (white arrow).

- High flow oxygen/humidified oxygen as necessary
- IV corticosteroid to reduce airway oedema
- IV antibiotics for penetrating injuries
- Manage oesophageal perforations with nasogastric (NG) tube/NBM and involvement of upper gastrointestinal (GI) surgeons as required

Operative

- Keep the patient NBM.
- If stable, get the informed consent from the patient by explaining benefits, risks and alternatives.
- Washout and closure (local anaesthetic) – superficial wounds not breaching platysma.
- Formal washout and exploration (general anaesthetic) – significant injuries or CT-confirmed vessel/organ injury (major trauma centre with vascular support).
- Surgical options during neck exploration can include:
  - Vessel repair/grafting – vascular input for arterial injury
  - Nerve repair
  - Organ repair
  - Tracheostomy
- Postoperative – close observations and serial examination may require repeat imaging and surgical re-exploration

Blunt injury

- Classify and manage extent of laryngeal trauma according to Schaefer's classification (Table 12.3)
- Non-operative adjuncts – anti-reflux medication, voice rest and SLT input

Table 12.3 Schaefer's classification and management of laryngeal injury from blunt neck trauma

Grade	Symptoms	Signs	Management
I	Minor airway symptoms	Minor endolaryngeal haematoma with no laryngeal fracture	Non-operative – observation, humidified oxygen, consider corticosteroids
II	Airway compromise	Laryngeal oedema and haematoma. Minor mucosal laceration. No exposed cartilage. Non-displaced laryngeal fracture	Panendoscopy with serial examination
III	Airway compromise	More significant laryngeal oedema and haematoma. Mucosal tears. Exposed cartilage. Displaced laryngeal fracture and vocal cord immobility	Panendoscopy. Tracheostomy is often required with surgical exploration and repair
IV	Airway compromise	Significant laryngeal oedema and haematoma. Severe mucosal tears. Unstable displaced laryngeal fracture and vocal cord immobility	Panendoscopy with tracheostomy, surgical exploration, repair and stent
V	Respiratory distress	Complete laryngo-tracheal separation	Emergency tracheostomy and repair through low cervical incision

Discharge and follow-up

- Discharge from hospital once all trauma-related injuries attended to and involved teams are satisfied
- ENT follow-up for laryngotracheal injuries

RED FLAGS

- High-impact trauma
- Symptoms and signs of airway compromise
- Hard signs of neck trauma on history and examination
- CT-confirmed vascular/organ injury
- Other trauma-related injuries

Chapter 13

Upper aerodigestive tract foreign body

Background

Aspiration or ingestion of foreign bodies (FB) in the upper aerodigestive tract is an ENT emergency and can be associated with significant morbidity and mortality. This may arise deliberately or accidentally and are more common in children than adults. Clinical presentation depends on the type, size and location of the FB. Upper airway FB can present acutely with respiratory distress, choking and stridor, whereas oesophageal FB often have a subacute presentation with dysphagia and odynophagia. It is critical to recognise any complications including airway obstruction, or oesophageal perforation with subsequent deep space neck collections/mediastinitis. For this chapter, we will focus on non-airway obstructing FBs as airway obstruction will be covered separately. Common sites of obstruction include the tonsils, tongue base, piriform fossae and the three classical narrowings of the oesophagus (cricopharyngeus, aortic arch and diaphragmatic hiatus). Management is dependent on patient factors and the type of FBs and may involve ENT, gastroenterology or general surgical teams depending on the site of obstruction and local clinician skill mix.

Potential areas of deterioration

A, B – risk of airway obstruction or aspiration of secretions/saliva
C – risk of oesophageal perforation with subsequent mediastinitis and septic shock

Preparation and equipment

- This is an ENT emergency, and the patient should be prioritised immediately.
- Attend the patient with headlight, tongue depressor, Tilley's or fish bone removal forceps and flexible nasendoscope.

History

Symptoms

- What did they eat? Clarify bone and type, button battery, sharp objects.
- When did they eat?
- Pain
- Able to eat and drink subsequently

DOI: 10.1201/b23238-17

- Can they localise with one finger where the FB sensation is?
- Measures employed to relieve symptoms so far.
- Previous similar episodes.

Systems

- Airway – difficulty in breathing, shortness of breath (SOB), aspiration/choking, drooling
- Oesophagus – dysphagia, odynophagia, regurgitation
- Voice – change in voice

Risk factors/red flags

- Chest pain radiating to the back
- Pyrexia
- Absolute dysphagia/odynophagia
- Recurrent food bolus obstruction may indicate oesophageal structural problem

AMPLE

- Allergies, regular/recent medications, other relevant past medical history, time of last meal

Examination

- Full ENT examination focussing on the oropharynx and laryngeal inlet.
- Neck – avoid palpating due to risk of dislodging any FB, assess range of motion and torticollis.
- Oropharynx – examine with headlight, especially tonsil and tongue base areas.
- FNE – look for obvious visible FB or signs suggestive of FB (pooling of saliva/food).
- Chest – palpation for surgical emphysema, auscultation for signs of aspiration.
- Full set of observations – signs of oesophageal perforation (tachycardia, tachypnoea, fever).

Management

Following confirmation of an FB in the upper aerodigestive tract and identification of its location, any FB can be either encouraged to pass medically or actively removed. Removal may be performed at the bedside under local anaesthetic or surgically under sedation/general anaesthetic. Sharp objects becoming lodged in the oesophagus or objects with a corrosive capacity (e.g. batteries) should be removed urgently.

Bedside removal

- Removal with forceps if FB visible in the oropharynx.
- Monitor for signs of bleeding post-removal.

Imaging

- Lateral soft tissue neck XR (Figure 13.1):
  - To locate radio-opaque FBs
  - Suggestive features of FB include loss of cervical lordosis or increased prevertebral soft tissue thickness (>0.5 vertebral body width above C4, or >1 below C4)

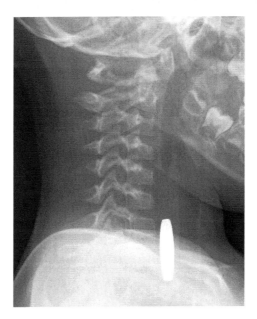

Figure 13.1 Lateral soft tissue neck X-ray image demonstrating a coin lodged in the oesophagus of a paediatric patient. There is also loss of cervical lordosis.

- CXR – features suggestive of oesophageal perforation (wide mediastinum, subcutaneous emphysema, pneumomediastinum)
- CT neck with contrast – to assess for radio-opaque FB or deep neck space collections

Conservative/medical

- If there is no convincing evidence of an FB, then patient may be managed conservatively – allow them to eat and drink and safety net patient to return if there are any further concerns.
- There is little evidence that carbonated drinks and hyoscine butylbromide (Buscopan) are more effective than a 'watch-and-wait' approach in the management of soft food boluses, but their use is widespread.

Surgical

- If medical management is ineffective then perform endoscopic removal using either rigid or flexible techniques (depending on site of obstruction and local policy).
- Keep the patient NBM.
- Informed consent of the patient by explaining benefits, risks and alternatives.
- Surgical options include removal
  - At induction by anaesthetist.
  - Rigid or flexible oesophagoscopy.
  - Rigid or flexible bronchoscopy.
- Examine oesophagus intra-operatively for signs of perforation and manage as below if any concerns.

Oesophageal perforation

- NBM and feed with NGT (placed intraoperatively under direct vision).
- Broad spectrum antibiotics.
- May need total parenteral nutrition (TPN) with a central line if unable to pass NGT.
- Reassess perforation with water soluble contrast swallow 7–10 days after the event.
- Surgical repair may be indicated after discussion with upper gastrointestinal team.

Discharge and follow-up

- Discharge patients if FB has been removed and no concerns regarding oesophageal perforation.
- Patients may benefit from 24 hours admission post procedure for monitoring for signs of perforation.
- No routine follow-up is required.

SIGNS OF OESOPHAGEAL PERFORATION

- Chest pain radiating to back
- Dysphagia
- Surgical emphysema
- Fever
- Tachycardia
- Tachypnoea

WHEN TO REFER FROM PRIMARY CARE

To ED
- Symptoms/signs of airway obstruction, oesophageal perforation

To emergency clinic
- Persistent symptoms of FB obstruction and dysphagia
- Patient concerns regarding FB with subacute history

Chapter 14

Deep space neck infections

Background

The structures of the neck are surrounded by layers of fascia. The superficial fascia contains the platysma muscle and is deep to the dermis. The muscles, vessels and viscera of the neck are surrounded by the deep cervical fascia, which can be further subdivided into three well-defined layers investing fascia, pretracheal fascia and prevertebral fascia, and the carotid sheath. Superficial veins, lymph nodes and cutaneous nerves are found in the space between the superficial and deep fascia (Figure 14.1). Within these fascial compartments are multiple deep neck spaces that communicate with each other. Some spaces extend down to the mediastinum, diaphragm and even as far as the coccyx. Deep neck spaces are clinically relevant as infection can easily spread quickly within these areas with significant associated morbidity and mortality (Table 14.1). Infections originating from the oral cavity, teeth, tonsils, face and superficial neck have the potential to progress to deep space neck infections. The local clinical signs of such infections result from the mass effect of pus, abscess cavity or inflamed tissue on surrounding structures. Management of these patients is focussed around early identification and resolution of the infective process either medically or surgically.

Potential areas of deterioration

A, B – risk of airway obstruction through external compression by large abscess/cavity
C – risk of septic shock

Preparation and equipment

• This is an ENT emergency, and the patient should be seen immediately.
• Attend the patient with headlight, tongue depressor, fibreoptic nasendoscope.

History

Symptoms

• Onset, timing and duration
• Laterality
• Better or worse

DOI: 10.1201/b23238-18

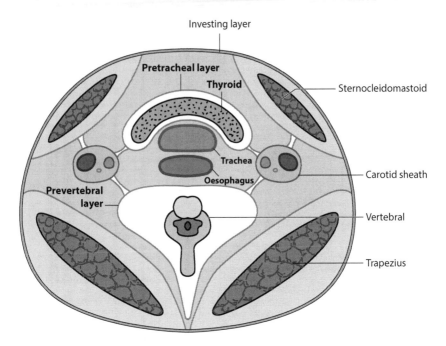

Figure 14.1 Diagram demonstrating the major contents of the neck in an axial plane as bound by the deep cervical fascia. This can be further subdivided into the investing fascia, pretracheal fascia and prevertebral fascia.

- Preceding symptoms – coryza, sore throat, tonsillitis, dental pain
- Previous episodes (especially those requiring hospital admission)
- Any treatment started prior to hospital

Systems

- Airway – difficulty in breathing, shortness of breath (SOB), aspiration/choking, drooling
- Oesophagus – dysphagia, odynophagia, regurgitation
- Voice – change in voice

Table 14.1 Complications of deep space neck infections

Airway	Oropharyngeal obstruction, external compression of trachea, rupture of cavity into trachea
Neck	Internal jugular vein thrombosis, carotid artery erosion, mycotic aneurysm, carotid blowout
Chest	Mediastinitis, empyema, pulmonary abscess
Cranial	Cranial nerve dysfunction, cerebral abscess
Osteomyelitis	Cervical spine, mandible, skull base
Systemic	Septic shock

Risk factors/red flags

- Recent dental work
- Chest/back pain
- Fever
- Rapid onset of SOB/difficulty in breathing, dysphagia/odynophagia, voice change
- Smoking, poor dental hygiene
- Immunocompromise

AMPLE

- Allergies, regular/recent medications, other relevant past medical history, time of last meal

Examination

- General inspection – toxic, sick, stable or unstable, drooling
- Respiratory distress – noisy breathing (stridor, stertor), tachypnoea, cyanosis, use of accessory muscles, anxiety, agitation, fatigue
- Mouth and oropharynx (Figure 14.2) – assess tonsils, peritonsillar spaces, trismus, uvula deviation, dental hygiene, raised floor of the mouth, palatal asymmetry
- Voice – speaking in full sentences, quality of voice, hoarseness, hot potato voice
- Neck – range of motion and torticollis, lumps, cellulitis, lymphadenopathy
- FNE – look for pooling of saliva, evidence of supraglottitis/epiglottitis, pharyngeal asymmetry/soft tissue bulge, inflammation and oedema of the glottis, vocal cord function
- Chest – auscultation for breath sounds
- Full set of observations – assess for signs of airway/breathing compromise (tachypnoea, reduced saturations) or sepsis (tachycardia, hypotension, fever)

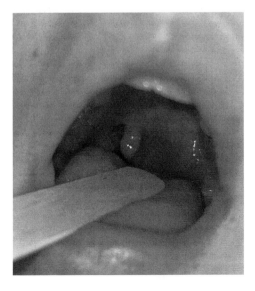

Figure 14.2 Clinical image of a left-sided quinsy (peritonsillar abscess).

Management

The principle of management in patients with deep space neck infections is clearance of the infection. This is usually medically with antibiotics, or surgical drainage. The principles of A to E resuscitation should be followed and early recognition and management of potential airway obstruction is essential. Medical management involves broad-spectrum antibiotics initially that can then be tailored according to microbiology results. In patients who are refractory to medical therapy, or those who present in a more moribund state, surgical intervention may be required. Surgical drainage can be performed externally or perorally depending on the site of the infection. Involvement of other members of the MDT may be required.

Bedside investigations

- Swab – mc&s
- Blood tests – FBC, U&Es, CRP, blood cultures, VBG with lactate

Imaging – to help localise infection and identify any spread/complications

- CT neck/chest with contrast (Figure 14.3)
  - localise infection, spread, complications
  - help plan any surgical intervention
  - presence of air indicates gas-forming organism
- MRI neck and chest – may provide improved soft tissue delineation
- CT angiogram – if suspicions of major neck vessel involvement
- Ultrasound – localise abscess cavity in the neck and help plan surgical intervention
  - USS-guided FNA to provide microbiology sample
- CXR – suggestive features of chest complications such as mediastinitis or pulmonary abscess

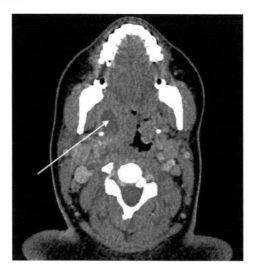

Figure 14.3 Axial CT neck demonstrating a fluid collection within the right parapharyngeal soft tissues with enhancing margins (white arrow). There is associated soft tissue swelling with consequent encroachment into the oropharyngeal airway.

Medical

- Antibiotics to cover likely polymicrobial causative organisms (aerobic and anaerobic).
    - IV is usually the route of choice.
    - Follow hospital antimicrobial policy for initial broad-spectrum choice.
- IV corticosteroid.
- IV fluids.
- Analgesia.

Surgical

- Keep the patient NBM.
- Informed consent of the patient by explaining benefits, risks and alternatives.
- Surgical options include:
    - Needle aspiration or incision and drainage of peritonsillar abscess.
    - External (transcervical) or peroral abscess drainage.

Discharge and follow-up

- Continue antibiotics with or without corticosteroids post-operatively with regular review.
- Monitor drain output from surgical drainage site and remove once minimal.
- Patients discharged with complete course of oral antibiotics.

RED FLAGS

- Signs of airway obstruction – stridor, inability to complete full sentences, increased respiratory effort, oxygen requirements
- Signs of severe infection – change in voice, limited neck movement, obvious external swelling, chest pain
- Signs of sepsis – toxic-looking patient, unstable, fever, tachycardia, hypotension

WHEN TO REFER FROM PRIMARY CARE

To ED
- Signs of airway obstruction
- Signs of severe infection
- Signs of sepsis
- Tonsillitis and unable to eat and drink

Chapter 15

Post-tonsillectomy bleed

Background

Tonsillectomy is a very commonly performed operation. While it is typically a straightforward day case procedure, development of a post-tonsillectomy bleed (PTB) is one of the leading risks. PTB can either be primary (within the first 24 hours of surgery) or secondary (after 24 hours of surgery). Estimates of PTB incidence are varied and are usually quoted to be around 1–2% for primary haemorrhage and 5–10% for secondary haemorrhage. PTB is more common in adolescent/young adult patients and for those patients whose procedure was performed for recurrent tonsillitis. The peak incidence of secondary haemorrhage is between days 5 and 7 post-operatively, although patients can present with significant bleeding at any point in the first 2 weeks. The mechanism behind primary haemorrhage is usually inadequate intraoperative haemostasis. With secondary haemorrhage, the likely trigger is significant post-operative pain and poor oral intake, leading to infection and subsequent bleeding. PTB should be taken seriously, especially in children who have a lower circulating blood volume than adults. Management is dependent on the severity of bleed and can sometimes result in a return to theatre.

Potential areas of deterioration

A, B – risk of airway obstruction or aspiration of blood
C – risk of haemorrhagic shock

Preparation and equipment

- This is an ENT emergency, and the patient should be seen immediately.
- Attend the patient with headlight, tongue depressor, swabs, 75% silver nitrate cautery sticks, adrenaline, Tilley's dressing forceps.

History

Operative history

- When was the procedure and in which hospital
- Bilateral/unilateral
- Indication
- Method used – cold steel, bipolar, coblation
- Any intraoperative or post-operative concerns prior to discharge

DOI: 10.1201/b23238-19

Symptoms

- Onset, timing and duration
- Frequency and number of episodes of bleeding
- Time since last bleed or actively bleeding
- Estimated quantity of blood loss
- Any preceding factors
- Pain post-procedure
- Managing to eat and drink

Systems

- Airway – difficulty in breathing, SOB, aspiration/choking, drooling
- Oesophagus – dysphagia, odynophagia, regurgitation
- Voice – change in voice

Risk factors/red flags

- Previous bleeding issues
- Known bleeding disorders (e.g. von Willebrand disease)
- Antiplatelet/anticoagulant medication
- Symptoms suggestive of large volume of blood loss – presyncope, loss of consciousness

AMPLE

- Allergies, regular/recent medications, other relevant past medical history, time of last meal

Examination

- Oropharynx (Figure 15.1) – examine with headlight assessing for signs of
  - Active bleeding or clots in the tonsillar fossae
  - Infection – erythematous, oedematous, excessively white sloughy tonsillar fossae

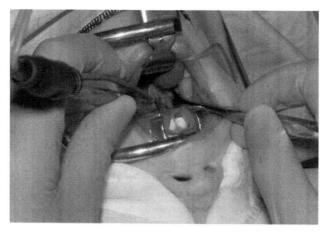

Figure 15.1 Intraoperative management of a post-tonsillectomy bleed with bipolar. A bleeding point is visible on the right tonsillar fossa.

- Oral cavity – teeth, lips, gums and temporomandibular joint (TMJ) for signs of damage or other bleeding points
- Flexible nasoendoscopy (FNE) – is not usually indicated but can be used if concerned about copious secretions and aspiration
- Chest – auscultation for signs of aspiration if appropriate
- Full set of observations – assess for signs of hypovolaemia (tachycardia, tachypnoea, hypotension)

Management

The principle of management in patients with a PTB is to stop the bleeding. Initial principles should follow resuscitation according to ALS/APLS principles. Paediatricians should be involved in the care of children with PTB. Patients can generally present in three categories:

1. Previous bleeding that has currently stopped
2. Minor bleeding that can be controlled non-operatively
3. Significant bleeding that needs a return to the operation theatre

Bedside investigations

- Blood tests – FBC, U&E, coagulation profile, group and save, cross match (if appropriate)

Previous bleeding that has currently stopped

- Assess level of pain and look for signs of infection.
- Admit the patient for close monitoring, IV antibiotics and analgesia to treat any secondary infection.
- Optimise analgesia – regular paracetamol, NSAIDs +/– opiates (if no contraindications)
- IV fluids for patients with dehydration
- Consider transfusion for patients who have significant anaemia secondary to blood loss

Minor bleeding

- Assess for a bleeding point with suction
- Stop bleeding with:
  - Direct pressure (swab, 1:10,000 adrenaline/tranexamic acid-soaked gauze held with Tilley's dressing forceps)
  - Silver nitrate cautery
- Medical adjuncts
  - IV tranexamic acid, antibiotics, IV corticosteroid
  - IV fluid
  - Optimise analgesia
  - Hydrogen peroxide gargles
- Topical haemostatic agents
  - Topical thrombin
  - Absorbable haemostatic agents – Floseal (thrombin/gelatin solution)
- Admit the patient for observation and keep them NBM as there is a risk of progressing to a significant bleed despite intervention

Major bleeding

- Keep the patient NBM.
- Informed consent of the patient/legal guardian by explaining benefits, risks and alternatives.
- Consider activation of major haemorrhage protocol.
- Surgical options include.
  - Bipolar diathermy.
  - Tie culpable vessel.
  - Underrun suture around bleeding area.
  - Pack tonsillar fossae with topical haemostatic agent (e.g. Surgicell) and suture fossae together.
  - Pack the tonsillar fossae and keep the patient intubated, transfer to ICU and relook the following day.

Discharge and follow-up

- Discharge patients if no evidence of further bleeding after 24 hours.
- Ensure haemoglobin is stable.
- Encourage patients to eat and drink.
- Discharge with oral antibiotics and analgesia.

RED FLAGS

- Signs of hypovolemic shock – tachycardia, hypotension
- Active torrential bleeding
- High-risk patients – child aged 11–17, bleeding diatheses, intraoperative complications

WHEN TO REFER FROM PRIMARY CARE

To ED
- Signs of active bleeding

Discuss with ENT
- Patients who have been complaining of active bleeding at home which is now controlled

Chapter 16

Post-thyroidectomy haematoma

Background

The surgical removal of the thyroid (thyroidectomy) is a procedure that is usually performed for refractory thyrotoxicosis, compressive multinodular goitre, or suspected/confirmed thyroid malignancy. While it is usually a safe procedure, there is a potential for the development of a post-operative haematoma. These usually occur within the first 24 hours after surgery. Even a small volume of haematoma can lead to airway obstruction and, therefore, it is vital to recognise this complication early. Management of these patients may be different to a typical emergency airway patient and often requires emergency bed-side intervention.

Potential areas of deterioration

A – risk of airway obstruction
C – risk of hypovolaemic shock if there is large active bleeding

Preparation and equipment

- This is an ENT emergency, and the patient should be seen immediately.
- Attend the patient with difficult airway trolley, flexible nasoendoscope, post-thyroid surgery emergency box (artery clip, scalpel, scissors, sterile gauze or medium wound pack, staple remover).
- Escalate to a senior ENT clinician and anaesthetist.

History

Symptom – pain, swelling

- Onset, timing and duration
- Better or worse
- Exacerbating or relieving factors
- Operative details – what procedure, indication, any other perioperative complications, abnormal anatomy, documentation of recurrent laryngeal nerve preservation, method of wound closure

Systems

- Airway – difficulty in breathing, SOB, aspiration/choking, drooling
- Oesophagus – dysphagia, odynophagia, regurgitation
- Voice – change in voice

DOI: 10.1201/b23238-20

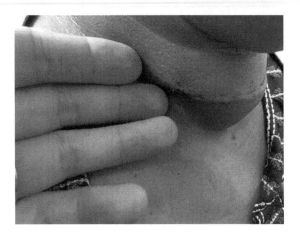

Figure 16.1 Clinical image of neck swelling following thyroidectomy representing haematoma.

Risk factors/red flags

- Known coagulopathy
- Long procedure with intraoperative complications

AMPLE

- Allergies, regular/recent medications, other relevant past medical history, time of last meal

Examination

- General inspection – agitation, anxiety, respiratory distress, stridor.
- Wound – dehiscence, discharge, erythema.
- Neck – palpate around wound to assess for swelling (fluctuant, boggy, hard, tender) (Figure 16.1), range of motion, torticollis.
- Drain – output, haematomas can still form in the presence of drains.
- Oropharynx – examine in full with headlight, any signs of swelling or bleeding.
- FNE – if there is an obvious haematoma compressing the airway then FNE may not be indicated, if there is a slower progression then look for signs of laryngeal oedema, swelling and vocal cord function.
- Full set of observations – assess for signs of respiratory distress (desaturation, tachypnoea).

Management

The principle of management in patients with post-thyroidectomy haematoma is early recognition and rapid haematoma evacuation. This to prevent airway obstruction through external tracheal compression. Patients should be monitored closely with a high index of suspicion for haematoma post-operatively. The following management steps highlight a stepwise approach. If the patient has improved and is stable after each step, then consider a planned return to theatre after discussion with the senior surgeon and anaesthetist.

Initial management

- High flow of oxygen (15 L/min through a non-rebreather mask)
- Head-up nursing

- Reassure and calm the patient
- Medical adjuncts – consider IV corticosteroid, IV tranexamic acid

Bedside haematoma evacuation

- Escalate to crash team/duty surgeon/most senior on-site anaesthetist
- Remove steristrips to expose the skin
- Cut skin sutures (usually subcuticular)
- Push fingers through the wound
- Open the skin
- Open the strap muscles (fingers or suture cutters)
- Evacuate the haematoma to expose the trachea
- Cover the wound with a (sterile/betadine soaked) pack

Local anaesthetic infiltration is not required prior to any of the above steps

- Open the strap muscles (fingers or suture cutters).
- Evacuate any haematoma formation to expose the trachea.
- Cover the wound with a betadine soaked or sterile pack.
- Local anaesthetic infiltration is not required prior to any of the above steps.

Return to theatre

- Unstable patient following bedside haematoma evacuation – emergency intubation (anaesthetist) and immediate return to theatre to evacuate the haematoma.
- Stable patient following bedside evacuation – return to theatre within 1–2 hours after consenting them and planning for a safe intubation and surgical approach.
- Return to theatre – haematoma evacuation and stopping any bleeding vessels (cautery, ties, clips).

Discharge and follow-up

- Discharge patients if they have been stable for 24–48 hours with no signs of haematoma recollection or other postoperative complications.
- Follow-up as per surgical pre-operative plan depending on indication for thyroid surgery.

RED FLAGS

- Key signs of post-thyroidectomy haematoma from early to late
  - Discomfort
  - Anxiety
  - Tachyponea
  - Difficulty in breathing
  - Difficulty in swallowing
  - Swelling
  - Stridor

Section II

Elective

Otology

Chapter 17

Hearing loss and audiology

Background

Hearing loss is a common presentation to ENT departments. Assessment begins with a thorough history, including the duration and progression of hearing loss over time. It is important to identify any preceding injuries or illnesses, as well as coexisting medical conditions that may represent the underlying cause of hearing loss (Table 17.1). Hearing loss can be divided into two categories, sensorineural hearing loss (SNHL) and conductive hearing loss (CHL). SNHL is more common, accounting for around 90% of cases. Sudden sensorineural hearing loss (SSNHL) is covered in detail in its own chapter. CHL occurs due to outer or middle ear dysfunction, whereas inner ear pathology results in SNHL. Bedside hearing tests such as tuning fork tests and free-field testing can help identify the type and severity of hearing loss. More sophisticated audiometry tests (e.g. Pure Tone Audiometry) provide an accurate assessment of hearing loss.

History

Symptoms

- Onset, timing and duration
- Laterality
- Course – stable, fluctuating, getting better or worse
- Previous episodes including previous treatments and their effects
- Precipitating factors – recent illness, trauma, noise exposure

Systems

- Ear – otalgia, otorrhoea, tinnitus, vertigo, facial weakness
- Neurology – slurred speech, limb weakness
- Autoimmune – rash, ulcers, myalgia, joint pain, dry mucous membranes

Past medical history

- Previous otological history and surgery
- Exposure to ototoxic medication
- History of autoimmune conditions
- Family history of hearing loss

DOI: 10.1201/b23238-23

Table 17.1 Causes of hearing loss

Conductive	Ear canal	Wax, foreign body, obstructive exostoses/osteoma, stenosis (congenital, post-inflammatory, radiotherapy)
	Tympanic membrane	TM perforation, extensive tympanosclerosis, retraction
	Middle ear	Glue ear, AOM, otosclerosis, ossicular discontinuity, eustachian tube dysfunction, glomus tumours
	Trauma	Temporal bone fractures, TM perforation
Sensorineural	Most common	Presbycusis, noise induced hearing loss
	Infection	Viral (Ramsay-Hunt syndrome, measles, mumps), bacterial (meningitis, syphilis)
	Inflammation	Labyrinthitis, Meniere's disease
	Malignancy	Vestibular schwannoma, other cerebellopontine angle tumours
	Drugs	Aspirin, loop diuretics, NSAIDs, aminoglycosides
	Trauma	Temporal bone fracture (otic capsule violating)
	Congenital	Infection (rubella, CMV, toxoplasmosis), syndromic hearing loss

Social history

- Occupation and associated importance of hearing
- Impact on quality of life, activities of daily living and hobbies

Examination

- Assess for functional signs of hearing loss – change in speech, difficulty in hearing conversation
- Inspection – pinna and mastoid process
- Otoscopy – evidence of external auditory canal (EAC) occlusion (e.g. wax, foreign body), otitis externa (OE), acute otitis media (AOM), glue ear, TM perforation
- Cranial nerves (especially facial nerve)
- Neurology – balance and gait
- Guided by the history, consider a systemic examination to identify systemic features of autoimmune conditions or vasculitis

Hearing tests

Free-field testing

- Quick, bedside test to screen for severity of hearing loss.
- Performed at 60 cm from the tested ear.
- Stand behind the patient to the tested side.

Table 17.2 Interpretation of free-field hearing tests

Voice level	Distance	Hearing
Whisper	60 cm	Normal
	15 cm	Mild loss
Conversational	60 cm	Mild/moderate loss
	15 cm	Moderate loss
Loud	60 cm	Severe loss

- Mask the non-test ear by rubbing the tragus.
- Whisper combination of 3 numbers and letters to the tested ear and ask the patient to repeat.
- If the patient unable to hear, then use whispered voice at 15 cm, progressing to conversational voice at 60 cm → conversational voice at 15 cm → loud voice at 60 cm.
- Interpretation of free-field hearing tests is summarised in Table 17.2.

Tuning fork tests

- Use a 512 Hz tuning fork – best balance between tone decay and vibrational sensation when testing air conduction (AC) versus bone conduction (BC).
- Interpretation of these results together allows to distinguish between CHL and SNHL.
- Rinne test:
  - Normally AC ≥ BC.
  - Strike the tuning fork and hold it 2–3 cm away from test ear and then directly on the mastoid tip, asking the patient which they hear loudest.
  - AC > BC (positive) suggests normal hearing or SNHL in the test ear.
  - BC > AC (negative) suggests CHL in the test ear.
- Weber test.
  - Distinguishes the affected ear.
  - Strike the tuning fork and place over vertex or mid-forehead.
  - In normal hearing, the sound should localise centrally.
  - In SNHL, the sound lateralises to the better hearing ear.
  - In CHL, the sound lateralises to the poorer hearing ear.

Pure tone audiometry (PTA) (Figure 17.1)

- Measures frequency-specific responses to different sound intensities (decibel hearing level – dB HL).
- Tones at specific frequencies are presented to each ear at different intensities (loudness) and patients are required to respond when they hear the tone.
- These responses are plotted to give a pictorial representation of their hearing.
- It measures both AC and BC responses (if AC is abnormal).

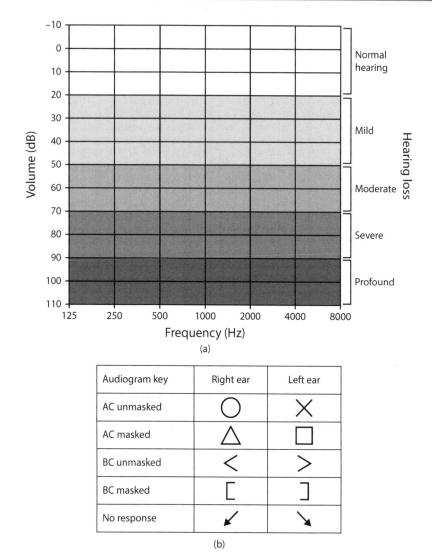

Figure 17.1 Baseline audiogram and its common symbols with hearing thresholds. (*Abbreviations:* AC: air conduction, BC: bone conduction.).

- Normal hearing is considered ≤ 20 dB HL.
- Figure 17.2 shows the appearance of CHL and SNHL on a pure tone audiogram

Tympanometry

- This is a measurement of acoustic impedance (flow of sound energy) through the middle ear.
- It provides information about middle ear function and health by virtue of sound reflected/transmitted by the middle ear.

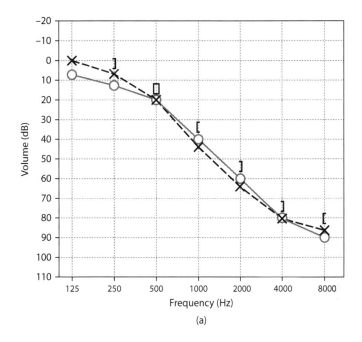

(a)

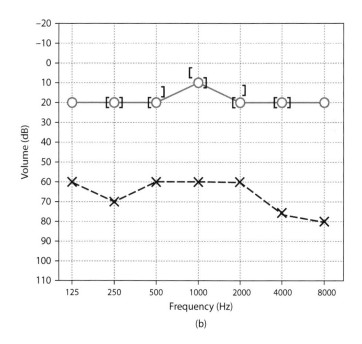

(b)

Figure 17.2 A PTA showing difference between CHL and SNHL. (a) Typical PTA as seen in presbyacusis (SNHL) showing a bilateral downsloping hearing loss pattern with no air bone gap. (b) Typical PTA showing a CHL pattern demonstrating a left-sided moderate loss.

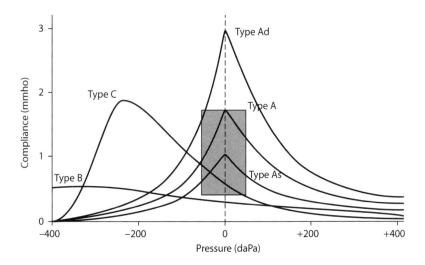

Figure 17.3 Different patterns seen on a tympanogram (type A, As, Ad, B, C).

- It also demonstrates middle ear compliance, middle ear pressure (daPa) and ear canal volume (mL).
- Figure 17.3 shows the appearance of different types of tympanogram.
- Table 17.3 summarises the common findings and interpretation of tympanometry.

Management

The principle in management of hearing loss is dependent on the type of loss, the underlying cause of hearing loss and the severity of hearing loss. Reversible causes such FB, wax impaction, otitis media with effusion (OME), otosclerosis should be individually assessed and treated accordingly. Broadly speaking, treatment is about

TABLE 17.3 Common findings and interpretation of tympanometry

Tympanometry type	Result and interpretation
Type A	Normal amplitude peak between −100 and +100 daPa
Type As	Shallow peak (reduced compliance) = stiff TM/ossicular chain (e.g. otosclerosis)
Type Ad	Tall peak (increased compliance) = flaccid TM (e.g. ossicular discontinuity)
Type B	Flat trace, no peak = non-mobile TM (e.g. OME or TM perforation)
Type C	Negative peak < −100 = negative middle ear pressure. May indicate eustachian tube dysfunction or mild OME

protecting residual hearing, empowering patients, and treating the underlying cause where possible, along with amplification with hearing aids.

Self-care and protection

- Keep ear clean and dry.
- Avoid trauma, e.g. use of cotton buds or itching the ear.
- Avoid loud noise exposure and wear protection where possible.

Conservative (rehabilitation)

- This includes hearing therapy to empower patients.
- Hearing aids.
  - There are a range of aids that can be offered depending on the severity and type of hearing loss.
  - These range from simple air conduction aids (usually behind-the-ear [BTE] type), bone conduction devices, and cochlear implants (reserved for bilateral profound hearing loss).

Surgical

- Surgery can be offered to patients where there is a rectifiable cause (CHL such as OME, otosclerosis or ossicular discontinuity).
- Patients need to be appropriately counselled of risks involved in surgery which include but are not limited to facial nerve injury, tinnitus, vertigo and worsening of hearing.
- Auditory implants may be utilised as part of the rehabilitation of hearing, such as bone-conduction hearing devices and cochlear implants.

Discharge and follow-up

- Patients with hearing loss can be either managed in the community or in secondary care depending on the type, cause and severity of their loss.
- This may be with the aid of audiologists and other members of the otology MDT.

RED FLAGS

- Sudden sensorineural hearing loss
- Asymmetric hearing loss
- Hearing loss following head trauma
- Referral otalgia
- History of Paget's disease – early treatment can minimise degree of loss

WHEN TO REFER FROM PRIMARY CARE

To emergency clinic/same-day discussion with ENT

- Sudden sensorineural hearing loss
- Unilateral hearing loss and facial weakness/altered sensation

- Hearing loss in immunocompromised patients with otalgia/otorrhoea (not responding after 72 hours of appropriate treatment)
- Hearing loss following head trauma – consider temporal bone fracture

To ENT clinic via cancer referral pathway

- Unilateral hearing loss/middle ear effusion can be a sign of nasopharyngeal carcinoma (more common in Southeast Chinese patients)

To otology clinic

- Hearing loss not explained by acute external/middle ear causes and not age-related
- Hearing loss associated with unilateral signs (e.g. tinnitus, vertigo)
- Asymmetrical hearing loss

Chapter 18

Otitis externa

Background

Otitis externa (OE) is a common condition in which there is inflammation of
any part of the external ear (pinna, EAC, outer surface of the TM) (Figure 18.1).
Infection is the most common aetiology; less frequently it can be caused by allergy
or irritation from underlying skin conditions, foreign body, or trauma. Infective OE
is most often caused by *Pseudomonas aeruginosa*, other Gram-negative organisms,
Staphylococcus aureus and *Streptococcus* species. Otitis externa can be subclassified
according to duration of symptoms: acute (less than 6 weeks, often bacterial
infection) or chronic (longer than 3 months, consider fungal infection) and
extent of disease: local or diffuse. Patients typically report itching, foul-smelling
discharge, pain and hearing loss. Examination findings may include swelling,
erythema and tenderness of the pinna, oedema of the EAC and mucopurulent
aural discharge. Necrotising otitis externa refers to extension of infection beyond
the external ear into the temporal bone/skull base and presents with deep-seated
severe otalgia, often in an elderly diabetic/immunocompromised patient
(see separate chapter).

History

Symptoms – itching/otorrhoea/pain/hearing loss

- Onset, timing and duration
- Laterality
- Severity of pain – controlled with analgesia or deep-seated otalgia causing difficulty
  in sleeping
- Characterise otorrhoea – purulent/blood-stained/odour/volume/consistency
- Exacerbating or relieving factors
- Previous episodes including previous treatments and their effects
- Trauma/triggers – e.g. cotton bud use/swimming

Systems

- Ear – otalgia, otorrhoea, tinnitus, vertigo, hearing loss, facial weakness
- Skin – pruritus, dry skin, pinna swelling/erythema
- Systemic – fever

DOI: 10.1201/b23238-24

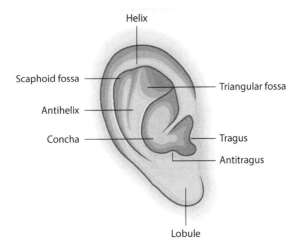

Figure 18.1 Pinna.

Past medical history

- Diabetes and control
- Skin conditions – eczema, contact dermatitis
- States of immunocompromise
- Previous ear surgery

Social history

- Smoking, alcohol status
- Performance status
- Impact on quality of life, activities of daily living and hobbies (e.g. swimming)

Examination

- General inspection and palpation of external ear – erythema, swelling, tragal tenderness
- Ear (Figure 18.2) – canal oedema, narrowing, erythema, debris, discharge, pain during speculum insertion, fungal hyphae, TM perforation, foreign bodies
- Facial nerve function

Management

The principle of management in patients with acute otitis externa is infection clearance. This is often with a combination of topical therapy and microsuction. Microbiology swabs are not usually required unless patients have recurrent/persistent OE. Topical ear drops provide a high antimicrobial concentration due to the small volume of the EAC, and thus have a very potent antibiotic effect that is often

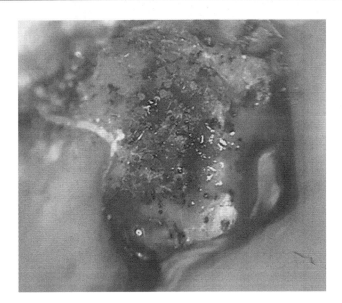

Figure 18.2 Clinical image of EAC with fungal infection (otomycosis).

independent of sensitivities. It is important to give patients aural care advice to prevent recurrence.

Self-care

- Keep ear clean and dry.
- Avoid trauma, e.g. use of cotton buds or scratching the ear.

Medical

- Topical ear drops/spray
  - Antibiotics – aminoglycosides (e.g. gentamicin) or quinolones (e.g. ciprofloxacin – preferred in cases of TM perforation)
  - Antifungals – e.g. clotrimazole
  - Combination antibiotic/antifungal with corticosteroids, e.g. Otomize, Sofradex
- Advise patients how to administer drops – lying flat during administration and for 5 minutes afterwards

Microsuction

- Aural toilet – clear debris, especially fungal hyphae if present, visualise TM and exclude perforation.
- Allows better delivery of medication to EAC.
- Ear wick insertion – canal oedema to allow delivery of medication, remove after 3–4 days.

Discharge and follow-up

- Patients can generally be discharged from clinic and do not require routine follow-up.

WHEN TO REFER FROM PRIMARY CARE

To emergency clinic
- Recurrent or persistent OE despite appropriate topical antibiotic therapy

Chapter 19

Acute otitis media

Background

Acute otitis media (AOM) is an infection of the middle ear which commonly affects young children between 3 months and 3 years of age. It is usually preceded by an upper respiratory tract infection followed by increasing otalgia and pyrexia, often evolving to mucopurulent ear discharge. Mostly, it is a self-limiting illness. However, if the illness is not improving after 72 hours, or the child displays features of significant systemic upset, antimicrobial treatment is advised. Complications arising from AOM can be significant and are broadly divided into intracranial and extracranial complications (Table 19.1).

History

Symptoms

- Onset and timing
- Sequence of events, e.g. URTI → otalgia → then mucopurulent otorrhoea
- Better or worse
- Exacerbating or relieving factors
- Previous episodes including previous treatments and their effects
- Trauma history

Systems

- Ear – otalgia, otorrhoea, tinnitus, vertigo, hearing loss, facial weakness
- Intracranial – nausea, vomiting, headache, loss of consciousness, seizures, rashes, features of meningism
- Change in child's behaviour – poor feeding, irritability, clumsiness
- Systemic features – fever, nausea, vomiting

Past medical history

- Paediatric primary immune deficiency (e.g. IgA deficiency, Di George syndrome)
- Cystic fibrosis/PCD
- Down's syndrome

Social history

- Parental smoking history
- Absence of breastfeeding

DOI: 10.1201/b23238-25

Table 19.1 Complications of AOM

Intracranial	Extracranial	
	Intratemporal	Extratemporal
Meningitis		
Cerebral abscess	Mastoiditis	Bezold's abscess (SCM)
Subdural abscess	Labyrinthitis (vertigo, hearing loss)	Citelli abscess (digastric fossa)
Epidural empyema	Facial nerve palsy	Luc abscess (temporal)
Sigmoid sinus thrombosis	Gradenigo syndrome (acute petrositis) – AOM, CN VI palsy, facial pain	Deep space neck abscess

- Nursery attendance
- Impact on school and quality of life

Risk factors/red flags

- Intracranial complication: Headaches, altered alertness, vomiting, swinging pyrexia
- Extracranial complication: Post-auricular swelling, diplopia (CN VI), facial nerve paralysis (CN VII)

Examination

- General inspection – pinna protruding and pushed forward, discharge, erythema
- Ear – bulging, red and hyperaemic TM, TM perforation (late phase, with debris in EAC) (Figure 19.1)

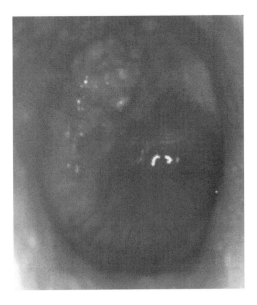

Figure 19.1 Endoscopic photograph of right tympanic membrane in acute otitis media.

- Mastoid – features of mastoiditis, e.g. post-aural fluctuant, erythematous and tender swelling (compared to contralateral side)
- Later phase may perforate with pulsatile discharge in EAC
- Examine other systems if suspecting complications:
  - Neurological – intracranial complications
  - Cranial nerves – facial nerve palsy, Gradenigo syndrome
  - Neck – extratemporal complications

Management

The principle of management in paediatric patients with AOM is to minimise pain symptoms and prevent complications

Investigations

- Swab – mc&s (if aural discharge and not responding to first line treatment)
- Bloods – FBC, U&E, CRP (if complicated AOM to monitor inflammatory markers)

Imaging

- Imaging is not routinely required unless concerned about intracranial or extracranial complications
- CT temporal bones – assess the mastoid air system
- CT head with contrast/MRI – assess for intracranial complications (Figure 19.2)
- CT neck with contrast – assess for neck collections (e.g. Bezold's abscess)

Conservative

- Most cases are viral, self-limiting and resolve within 72 hours.

Medical

- Analgesia (topical or systemic)
- Antibiotics if systemically unwell or not improving after 72 hours (usually penicillin)
- Febrile children <3 months or when suspecting a complication – seek urgent paediatric attention

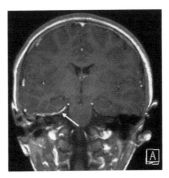

Figure 19.2 Coronal contrast-enhanced MRI of a child with otogenic meningitis (arrow indicating rural enhancement).

Surgical

- Not utilised in uncomplicated episodes of AOM
- Myringotomy and ventilation tube insertion in cases of recurrent AOM

Discharge and follow-up

- Patients are usually managed in primary care or in outpatients and do not need routine follow-up.
- For complicated AOM requiring admission/surgery, patients can be discharged when apyrexial on oral antibiotics and followed-up in ENT clinic to assess for complete resolution.

RED FLAGS

- Febrile child <3 months
- No improvement after 24–48 hours of antibiotics
- Suspicions of complications (neurological involvement, swinging fevers, vertigo, hearing loss, mastoid/SCM/digastric/temporal swellings)

WHEN TO REFER FROM PRIMARY CARE

To ED
- Suspicions of AOM with complications

To emergency clinic
- Failure to resolve despite treatment

To routine otology clinic
- Persistent perforation
- >6 attacks a year for more than one year

Chapter 20

Cholesteatoma

Background

Cholesteatoma is a non-malignant but destructive and locally invasive disease of abnormal desquamated keratinised cells and squamous debris. They typically originate in the middle ear cleft and rarely from the external auditory canal (EAC). Cholesteatomas can be divided into congenital or acquired. Congenital cholesteatoma is a rare disease of children that is believed to be a result of trapped squamous epithelium or metaplasia during embryological development. It is diagnosed from a pearly white mass behind an intact TM in a child with a conductive hearing loss. Acquired cholesteatoma is much more common and has an unclear pathogenesis. It is presumed to be a consequence of eustachian tube dysfunction and chronic inflammation following repeated middle ear disease, or following TM injury secondary to acute otitis media, trauma or otological surgery. Patient groups with higher incidences of cholesteatoma formation include patients with cleft palate and some syndromes such as Treacher-Collins, Downs, and Turners. It is important to be able to recognise cholesteatoma as untreated disease can leave the locally destructive process unchecked. Potential complications within the temporal bone include recurrent infection, hearing loss (secondary to TM/ossicular chain destruction or cochlear involvement), facial nerve palsy and vertigo due to a labyrinthine fistula. There is also the risk of extra-temporal and intracranial complications as with acute otitis media. Following surgical management, there can be a 10–15% chance of disease recurrence and a 5–10% chance of disease developing in the contralateral ear.

History

Symptoms – patients commonly present with recurrent otorrhoea or hearing loss

- Onset, timing and duration
- Laterality
- Frequency of discharge, number of episodes, response to topical antibiotics
- Severity of subjective hearing loss, especially between infections
- Prior history of recurrent ear infections (OE or OM)
- Preceding trauma

Systems

- Ear – otalgia, bloody otorrhea, tinnitus, vertigo, hearing loss, facial weakness

DOI: 10.1201/b23238-26

Past medical history

- Cleft palate
- Otological surgery
- Congenital abnormalities if it is a child
- Diabetes or other immunosuppression

Social history

- Smoking, alcohol status
- Performance status
- Impact on quality of life, activities of daily living and hobbies

Examination

- General inspection of external ear – active discharge, erythema
- Otoscopy/microscope (Figure 20.1) – canal wall defect, aural polyp, attic abnormality (crust, keratin debris, bony erosion), TM retraction/perforation
- Facial nerve status
- Neurological – if there are concerns regarding intracranial complications

Management

The principle of management in cholesteatoma is to maintain a safe, dry ear. This can be achieved through non-operative or surgical approaches. It is important to perform a thorough workup in order to evaluate the extent of disease, as this will influence choice of management. As cholesteatoma can present in a variety of ways, this will also help identify what is concerning the patient the most so that a tailored management plan can be discussed.

Bedside investigations

- Ear swab – mc&s
- Biopsy – aural polyp, granulation tissue

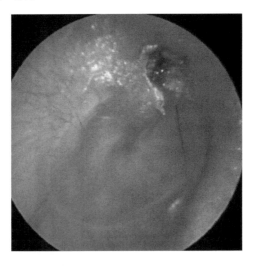

Figure 20.1 Endoscopic photograph of right attic (pars flaccida) cholesteatoma.

- Audiometry – differentiate between conductive and sensorineural hearing loss
- Blood tests – FBC, U&E, CRP (not always indicated)

Imaging – cholesteatoma is usually a clinical diagnosis but imaging is useful for excluding other differentials and helping to plan for surgery if indicated

- CT temporal bones to assess
  - extent of disease
  - integrity of middle and inner ear structures (ossicular chain, otic capsule and facial nerve)
- Non-EPI diffusion-weighted MRI – residual disease, recurrence

Non-operative

- Regular microsuction and clearance to decompress cholesteatoma sac
- Treat recurrent infections with topical drops as per OE medical management

Surgical

- Canal wall up (combined approach tympanoplasty)
- Canal wall down (atticotomy or modified radical mastoidectomy)
- The differences between canal wall up and canal wall down procedures are highlighted in Table 20.1

Discharge and follow-up

- Patients with canal wall down procedures and a long-term cavity may require regular outpatient review for cavity care compared to those with a canal wall up procedure.

RED FLAGS

- Facial palsy
- Vertigo
- Signs of intracranial extension

Table 20.1 Difference between canal wall up and canal wall down procedures

Canal wall up	Canal wall down
Normal EAC anatomy preserved	Associated with a cavity
Multi-stage procedure	Single-stage procedure
Self-cleaning cavity (useful due to less post-operative care and clinic visits, e.g. in paediatrics)	Often requires regular post-operative care and clinic reviews for microsuction and cavity cleaning
Better hearing outcomes	Poorer average hearing outcomes
Higher risk of residual disease and recurrence – may require more regular imaging	Reduced chance of residual disease and recurrence

WHEN TO REFER FROM PRIMARY CARE

To ED
- Complications of cholesteatoma – facial palsy, vertigo, signs of intracranial extension

To emergency clinic
- Non-resolving/recurrent ear discharge – more likely to represent recurrent OE
- Unexplained asymmetrical hearing loss – may represent sudden sensorineural hearing loss

To otology clinic
- Suspicion of cholesteatoma (chronic foul-smelling discharging ear, hearing loss, signs suggestive of cholesteatoma on examination)

Chapter 21

Dizziness and vertigo

"Dizziness" is a common descriptive term used by patients to describe a variety of sensations. ENT causes of imbalance tend to result in vertigo; this is the illusion of movement, usually an experience of spinning or one's surroundings or oneself. It is, therefore, important to pinpoint the patient's description of dizziness to distinguish true vertigo from similar symptoms such as unsteadiness, light-headedness or blackouts. Normal balance function is dependent on sensory information input from the vestibular, visual and proprioceptive systems. These inputs are processed in the central nervous system to allow visuo-spatial awareness, through gaze and postural control. A defect in any of the sensory or central systems can present as dizziness or vertigo. Central causes that should be considered include posterior circulation stroke, posterior fossa space occupying lesions, and migraine. Sensory inputs from the peripheral vestibular apparatus (semi-circular canals and otolith organs) work alongside visual stimuli to generate a normal vestibulo-ocular reflex. Key differences in the history, such as triggers and duration, and examination, can help distinguish between peripheral and central causes of vertigo (Table 21.1). The common causes of vertigo-associated features are summarised in Table 21.2. The most common causes of vertigo are benign, but the symptoms can be highly intrusive and have an adverse impact on quality of life. Therefore, understanding the principle causes and features of vertigo is paramount to providing the correct management.

History

Symptoms

- Establish true vertigo versus other dizzy sensations
- Onset, duration and timing
- Frequency of episodes
- Triggers, e.g. head movement in BPPV, loud noises in SSCD
- Relieving factors
- Preceding illness, e.g. viral disease in acute peripheral vestibular loss
- Trauma history (to ear or head)
- Intrusive nature, e.g. present day and/or night, impact on sleep
- Coping strategies
- New medications

DOI: 10.1201/b23238-27

Table 21.1 Factors that can aid distinguishing between peripheral and central vertigo

Domain	Peripheral	Central
Onset	Sudden onset, intermittent vertigo	Gradual onset, persistent vertigo
Symptom severity	Severe vertigo	Milder vertigo, can be severe in stroke
Triggers	Head position/movement	Minimal (vertigo is more constant)
Nausea and vomiting	Frequent and often severe	Less predictable
Nystagmus direction	Unidirectional, usually horizontal/torsional	Vertical, multidirectional, downbearing
Hearing loss/tinnitus	Can be present	Less likely
Motor function, gait, coordination	Typically normal	Can be affected

Systems

- Ear – otalgia, otorrhoea, tinnitus, hearing loss, ear fullness, unilateral signs
- Neurological – presyncope, syncope, headaches +/– aura, loss of consciousness, seizures, facial numbness or pain
- Visual – change in vision, pain on eye movement, photo/phonophobia
- Systemic features – nausea, vomiting, weight loss

Past medical history

- Viral or bacterial illness, e.g. COVID-19 infection, meningitis, upper respiratory tract
- Risk factors for stroke, e.g. cardiovascular disease

Table 21.2 Common causes and features of vertigo

Peripheral	Benign positional paroxysmal vertigo (BPPV) – vertigo lasts seconds, typically on turning in bed/looking up or down
	Vestibular neuronitis (vertigo with normal hearing) – days to weeks
	Labyrinthitis (hearing loss, vertigo) – days to weeks
	Meniere's disease (hearing loss, vertigo, tinnitus, and aural fullness) – hours
	Superior semi-circular canal dehiscence syndrome (SSCD) – seconds to minutes, may be triggered by loud sounds (Tullio phenomenon)
	Vestibular migraine – hours to days
	Vestibular schwannoma – chronic
	Ear pathology – otitis externa, otitis media, eustachian tube dysfunction
	Drugs – Aminoglycosides, aspirin, loop diuretics, NSAIDs, macrolides
Central	Posterior circulation stroke
	Multiple sclerosis
	Cerebellar tumours
	Vestibular migraine
	Head trauma

- Migraine
- Previous middle ear disease
- Ear surgery/neurosurgery
- Radiotherapy exposure
- Psychiatric conditions

Drug history

- Recent, current and over-the-counter medication, e.g. anticonvulsants

Social history

- Smoking, alcohol status
- Performance status
- Impact on quality of life and activities of daily living
- Job and nature of work (e.g. working at height, professional driver)

Family history

- Hearing loss, Neruofibromatosis type 2 (NF2)

Examination

- General inspection of pinna – discharge, erythema
- Otoscopy – cholesteatoma, OE, OM, TM (perforation, sclerosis, vascular lesion, glomus tumour)
- Neurological – full cranial nerve examination (facial nerve palsy), Rinne's and Weber's test, cerebellar examination, gait examination
- Special tests
  - Dix-Hallpike – assess for BPPV
    - Patient keeps eyes open and looking forward with head tilted to 45 degrees
    - Lie patient down rapidly with support to extend their head 20 degrees over the end of the bed
    - Observe the eyes for nystagmus – latency, torsional/rotational, fatigable
    - Care in patients with neck problems or carotid sinus syncope
  - Head impulse test – assess unilateral peripheral vestibular hypofunction
    - Patient is advised to fix their gaze on the examiner's nose and the head is rapidly turned to one side while watching the eyes for presence of any corrective catchup saccadic eye movements
  - Unterberger's test – assess labyrinthe pathology
    - Patient closes eyes and marches on the spot
    - Positive test = lateral rotation >30 degrees towards the affected labyrinth
  - Romberg's test – assess truncal proprioception
    - Patient stands upright with their eyes closed
    - Positive test = patient falls
  - HINTS exam for acute vertigo – comprises three components that helps to differentiate between peripheral (e.g. vestibular neuronitis) and central (stroke) vertigo (Table 21.3):
    - Head impulse test to assess vestibulo-ocular reflex (VOR)
    - Nystagmus
    - Test of Skew (alternate cover test)

Table 21.3 Interpretation of HINTS examination

	Peripheral	Central
Head impulse test	Positive – loss of eye fixation with head movement	Negative – normal eye fixation and thus intact VOR
Nystagmus	None, horizontal, unidirectional	Vertical, rotatory or bidirectional
Test of skew	Negative – Absent skew	Positive – present skew

Management

The principles of management are led by the underlying cause, symptom severity and patient choice. Much of the diagnosis can be obtained through a thorough history and examination. Therefore, the following investigations listed are useful for select cases only when a specific cause of vertigo is suspected. Conservative management includes vestibular rehabilitation to help restore balance function through education and a programme of head, neck and eye exercises. Medications including antihistamines (cyclizine, promethazine) or antipsychotics (prochlorperazine) can be used to help alleviate symptoms of vertigo and associated nausea. These should only be used for a short period to allow the body's normal vestibular compensatory mechanisms to work.

Bedside investigations

- PTA +/– tympanograms +/–stapedial reflexes.
- Blood tests are not usually indicated.
- Caloric, VEMP (vestibular evoked myogenic potential testing) and rotational chair testing may be arranged in specific cases.

Imaging

- MRI IAM/brain – cerebellopontine angle tumours

Conservative

- Education – trigger avoidance.
- Lifestyle measures – avoid caffeine, chocolate, alcohol, smoking, salt (especially in Meniere's disease/vestibular migraine).
- Vestibular rehabilitation for central compensation (e.g. Cawthorne-Cooksey exercises).
- Particle-repositioning manoeuvres (e.g. Epley manoeuvre – for BPPV (Figure 21.1)).
  - This is a continuation of the Dix-Hallpike test where the head is rotated a further 90 degrees followed by turning the head and body over onto the opposite shoulder then sitting up.
- Home exercises, e.g. Brandt-Daroff for BPPV.
- Hearing support if hearing affected.
- Driving avoidance if there is sudden onset of vertigo without warning.

Medical

- Short-term antiemetics – cyclizine, promethazine
- Short-term vestibular sedatives – prochlorperazine, benzodiazepines

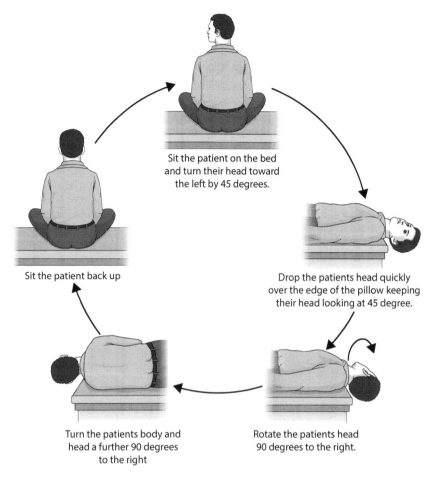

Sit the patient on the bed
and turn their head toward
the left by 45 degrees.

Sit the patient back up

Drop the patients head quickly
over the edge of the pillow keeping
their head looking at 45 degree.

Turn the patients body and
head a further 90 degrees
to the right

Rotate the patients head
90 degrees to the right.

Figure 21.1 **Steps of the Epley manoeuvre.**

- Meniere's disease – consider betahistine, bendroflumethiazide or intratympanic corticosteroids
- Prophylactic migraine treatment in vestibular migraine

Surgical

- Meniere's disease – endolymphatic sac surgery, micropressure therapy, vestibular nerve section, labyrinthectomy
- Vestibular schwannoma – stereotactic radiotherapy, microsurgical excision

Discharge and follow-up

- Patients with vertigo can usually be managed on an outpatient basis.

RED FLAGS

- Signs and symptoms of central vertigo
- Unliteral ear signs
- Severe vertigo contributing to falls risk

WHEN TO REFER FROM PRIMARY CARE

To ED
- ENT referral – cranial nerve (CN) or facial nerve palsy
- Neurological referral – focal neurological signs

Routine
- Persisting symptoms despite primary care management, e.g. BPPV, acute vestibular failure
- Suspected conditions:
  - Meniere's disease
  - Vestibular schwannoma
- Neurology/ENT referral in suspected vestibular migraine

Chapter 22

Tinnitus

Background

Tinnitus is a commonly reported symptom which has many underlying causes; in some cases, it can cause great distress for patients. It is usually the false perception of sound in the absence of an external stimulus but, rarely, can be objective with an internal sound source. Subjective tinnitus is most often non-pulsatile and typically described as a ringing, hissing or humming sound. For some patients, tinnitus can be extremely intrusive, generating great upset and negatively impacting on their well-being. It can frequently coexist alongside mental health conditions and, therefore, consultations require patience, understanding and a support environment. Due to the numerous potential underlying causes (Table 22.1), it is important to obtain a thorough history as this will help identify the minority of patients that require further investigations. The pathophysiology of subjective tinnitus is not clearly understood, but proposed theories include dysfunction in the processing of sounds in the cortical auditory pathways, genetic risk factors and cochlear irregularities. Treatment is usually conservative, but medical and, very rarely, surgical options may be required, depending on the cause.

History

Symptoms

- Onset, timing and duration
- Characterise sound – type and pulsatility
- Bilateral or unilateral (laterality)
- Better or worse
- Exacerbating or reliving factors
- Preceding trauma, including barotrauma
- Intrusiveness – present day and/or night, impact on sleep
- Coping strategies trialled
- New medications

Systems

- Ear – otalgia, otorrhoea, vertigo, hearing loss, facial weakness, unilateral signs
- Neurological – presyncope, loss of consciousness, headache

DOI: 10.1201/b23238-28

Table 22.1 Causes of tinnitus

Subjective tinnitus	
Idiopathic	Most common
Ear	Hearing loss, e.g. presbycusis, noise-induced, barotrauma, Ménière's disease
Brainstem	Cerebellopontine angle lesion (vestibular schwannoma, meningioma)
Neurological	Meningitis, head trauma, multiple sclerosis, cerebellar disease
Metabolic	Diabetes mellitus, thyroid disease, hyperlipidaemia
Psychological	Anxiety, depression, stress
Medication (ototoxic)	Aminoglycosides, NSAIDs, loop diuretics, salicylates
Objective tinnitus	
Vascular	Arteriovenous malformations, carotid stenosis, benign intracranial hypertension, hypertension, high jugular bulb, middle ear tumours, persistent stapedial artery
Neuromuscular	Middle ear myoclonus, e.g. stapedial, tensor tympani
Other	Patulous eustachian tube

Abbreviation: NSAIDs, nonsteroidal anti-inflammatory drugs.

Past medical history

- Diabetes
- Hypertension
- Meningitis
- Previous middle ear disease
- Ear or head surgery
- Radiotherapy to the head
- Psychiatric conditions – including any current suicidal thoughts
- Family history of hearing loss

Social history

- Smoking, alcohol status
- Impact on quality of life, activities of daily living and hobbies
- Job and nature of work, e.g. exposure to loud noise, headphones, earphones

Examination

- General inspection of pinna – discharge, erythema
- Otoscopy – cholesteatoma, otitis externa (OE), otitis media (OM), tympanic membrane (TM) (perforation, sclerosis, vascular lesion, glomus tumour)
- Neurological – full cranial nerve examination, cerebellar examination
- Auscultate for bruits in the neck, temporal and mastoid areas
- Hearing – tuning fork, free-field hearing test

Management

The principle of management in patients with tinnitus is dependent on the underlying cause. The management for subjective non-pulsatile tinnitus often requires a multidisciplinary approach which is involves psychological therapies, such as tinnitus retraining therapy, and improving coping strategies. Cognitive behavioural therapy is also used in cases of highly intrusive tinnitus. In addition to psychological therapies, devices to help mask sound and hearing aids (if underlying hearing loss) can be used. Management options for objective tinnitus can be either medical and/or surgical. Medical strategies can include blood pressure control in vascular causes such as AV malformations with or without surgical input. Intracranial pathology such as tumours will require neurosurgical advice and management.

Bedside investigations

- Pure tone audiometry (PTA) with or without tympanograms and stapedial reflexes
- Blood tests (rarely needed) – FBC, U&E, TFT, HbA1c, Lipid profile, Syphilis serology

Imaging

- MRI IAM/brain – cerebellopontine angle tumours
- CT angiogram – pulsatile/objective tinnitus
- Carotid doppler

Subjective tinnitus

- Conservative
  - Tinnitus retraining therapy
  - CBT
  - Distracting techniques – with added environmental sounds, e.g. television, radio, tinnitus apps
  - Relaxation – including hypnosis
  - Support groups
  - Hearing aids – if hearing loss
  - Masking devices, e.g. white noise generators
- Medical – little evidence for efficacy and no specific licensed medication
  - Glutamate receptor antagonists – e.g. acamprosate
  - GABA receptor agonists – e.g. benzodiazepines
- Surgical – less common and usually reserved for subjective tinnitus with hearing loss
  - Stapedotomy, e.g. in otosclerosis
  - Middle ear implants for conductive hearing loss
  - Cochlear implants in SNHL
  - Microvascular decompression, e.g. trigeminal neuralgia

Objective tinnitus

- Conservative – relaxation/distraction strategies
- Medical
  - Anti-hypertensive medication for vascular causes and hypertension
  - Muscle relaxants for myoclonus

- Surgical
    - ENT – tympanotomy and division of middle ear tendon in myoclonus, excision of middle ear vascular tumours (glomus tympanicum)
    - Vascular – embolisation of AV malformation, carotid endarterectomy in carotid stenosis
    - Neurosurgical – intracranial tumour removal

Discharge and follow-up

- Patients with tinnitus can usually be managed on an outpatient basis.

RED FLAGS

- Unilateral tinnitus
- Pulsatile tinnitus
- Sudden onset tinnitus
- Associated asymmetrical hearing loss
- Associated significant vertigo
- Associated neurology
- Psychological distress/suicidal ideation

WHEN TO REFER FROM PRIMARY CARE

Urgent/same day

- ENT referral – CN or facial nerve palsy
- Neurosurgical referral – focal neurological signs
- Psychiatry – suicidal ideation

ENT emergency clinic

- Microsuction – wax
- FB removal
- Persisting infection

Routine

- Bilateral/unilateral/pulsatile tinnitus with non-urgent features

Chapter 23

Facial nerve palsy

Background

The facial nerve (seventh cranial nerve) is a mixed nerve comprising upper and lower motor neurons, as well as motor and sensory fibres. It originates in the pons and travels through the cerebellopontine angle to the internal acoustic meatus. The nerve traverses the temporal bone within the facial canal, where it provides three branches (greater superficial petrosal to the lacrimal gland, nerve to stapedius and chorda tympani supplying taste to the anterior two-thirds of the tongue), before exiting the cranium through the stylomastoid foramen, giving a further three branches (posterior auricular nerve and nerves to posterior belly of the digastric and stylohyoid muscles). Finally, the nerve terminates within the parotid gland in five named branches (temporal, zygomatic, buccal, marginal mandibular and cervical) which supply the muscles of facial expression (Figure 23.1). Patients with a facial nerve palsy most commonly present with facial asymmetry due to weakness of these muscles (Figure 23.2). There may also be more subtle symptoms/signs due to involvement of other branches, such as hyperacusis, or changes in taste or tear production.

ENT doctors are involved in managing patients with peripheral (lower motor neuron) facial nerve palsies. The muscles of the forehead are innervated bilaterally at the brainstem level so in central (upper motor neuron) lesions there is sparing of these muscles. There are many causes of peripheral facial nerve weakness (Table 23.1); however, 80% of cases are attributed to Bell's (idiopathic) palsy. Bilateral facial nerve palsy is rare and should raise suspicions for underlying neurological disease such as Guillain-Barre syndrome, Lyme disease or syphilis. The incidence of Bell's palsy is estimated to be between 20 and 30 cases per 100,000 people per year, with an 8% chance of recurrence. Bell's palsy is a diagnosis of exclusion and care should be taken to ensure that other causes of facial nerve palsy are identified and investigated appropriately. The majority of patients will show some recovery within 3 weeks with or without treatment. The mainstay of management in patients with facial nerve palsy is identification of any underlying cause, and prompt treatment to reduce the risk of long-term paralysis.

History

Symptoms

- Onset, timing and duration
- Laterality

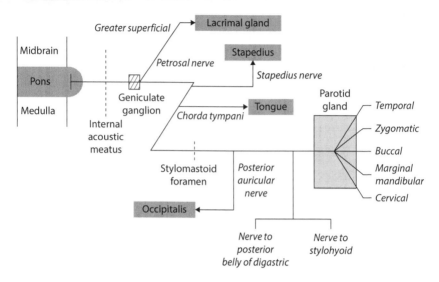

Figure 23.1 The anatomy of the facial nerve through its course including its motor and sensory branches and the structures they supply.

- Progression
- Previous similar episodes
- Trauma history
- Ability to close eye
- Synkinesis (development of linked or unwanted facial movements), hemifacial spasm, pain
- Effect on ability to eat/drink, speech, taste, tear production, hearing

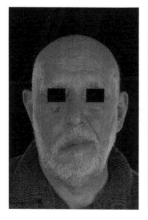
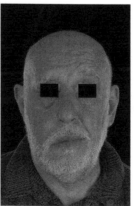
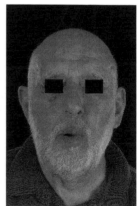

Figure 23.2 Clinical photographs of patient with facial nerve palsy. (Courtesy of Mr. Charlie Huins.)

Table 23.1 Causes of facial nerve palsy

Idiopathic	Bell's palsy (diagnosis of exclusion)
Ear	Otitis media, cholesteatoma, Ramsay-Hunt syndrome, necrotising otitis externa
Neck/face	Parotid disease (usually malignant with perineural invasion), facial nerve schwannoma
Brainstem	Cerebellopontine angle lesion (vestibular schwannoma, meningioma)
Infection	Diabetes mellitus, Lyme disease, Guillain-Barre syndrome, HIV, EBV, CMV
Trauma	Temporal bone fracture, middle ear/temporal bone/ parotid surgery (iatrogenic)
Congenital	Mobius syndrome, CHARGE syndrome
Upper motor neuron	Stroke, cerebral aneurysm, multiple sclerosis, intracranial infection, cerebral tumours

Systems

- Ear – otalgia, otorrhoea, tinnitus, vertigo, hearing loss
- Parotid – swelling, lump, pain
- Neurological – exclude symptoms suggestive of central lesions (slurred speech, visual disturbance, limb weakness, symptoms of intracranial infection)

Past medical history

- Poorly controlled diabetes
- Current pregnancy
- Immunocompromise
- Previous temporal bone/middle ear/parotid surgery
- Congenital abnormalities (if patient is a child)

Social history

- Smoking, alcohol status
- Performance status
- Impact on quality of life, activities of daily living and hobbies

Examination

- Facial nerve – general inspection for asymmetry, drooling, grade palsy according to House-Brackmann scale (Table 23.2)
    - Temporal – raise eyebrows (examining frontalis muscle)
    - Zygomatic – close eyes (orbicularis occuli)
    - Buccal – puff out cheeks (buccinator), show teeth (orbicularis oris)
    - Marginal mandibular – show teeth, pout (mentalis)
    - Cervical – platysma
- Eye – effort to close, evidence of corneal abrasion if unable to close

Table 23.2 House-Brackmann scale for grading facial nerve palsies

Grade	Description
I	Normal facial nerve function
II	Slight weakness noticeable with movement, normal tone and function at rest
III	Able to close eye with effort, obvious weakness/ asymmetry but not disfiguring
IV	Inability to close eye, disfiguring weakness/asymmetry
V	Obvious asymmetry at rest, barely perceptible movement
VI	Complete paralysis with no movement

- Ear – general inspection (discharge, erythema), otoscopy (cholesteatoma, OM, vesicles, granulation tissue, polyps)
- Parotid – examination for masses
- Facial rashes/vesicles
- Oral cavity – palatal weakness and vesicles
- Neurological – full cranial nerve and limb examination

Management

The principle of management in facial nerve palsy is to identify any cause, treat this specifically, and minimise the risk of any long-term paralysis. Much of the diagnosis can be obtained through a thorough history and examination. Therefore, the investigations listed next are useful for select cases when suspecting a specific cause of facial nerve palsy and should not be ordered as a blanket workup for all patients. Patients should be counselled regarding the risk of incomplete resolution with initial therapy, which may later require facial rehabilitation therapy, botulinum toxin injections or delayed surgical interventions (to try and improve muscle tone, facial expression and synkinesis).

Bedside investigations

- Ear swab – mc&s if ear discharge
- PTA (+/– tympanograms and stapedial reflexes)
- Blood tests – FBC, U&E, CRP, viral serology

Imaging

- USS +/– FNAC – parotid masses
- CT temporal bones – cholesteatoma, necrotising otitis externa
- MRI brain – cerebellopontine angle tumour
- CT head – upper motor neuron causes

Special tests – not frequently used in clinic settings

- Schirmer's test – for tear production
- Formal taste testing – salt, sweet, bitter
- Salivary flow testing

Bell's palsy medical management

- Commence 'high-dose' oral coticosteroids (prednisolone) after discussing the risks and benefits with the patient.
- Oral prednisolone dosing regimens are variable, an example is:
  - 1 mg/kg (max 60 mg) for 7 days then tapered by 10 mg per day.
- Demonstrated benefit only with early treatment (<72 hours).
- Antivirals can be added if Ramsay-Hunt syndrome.
- 85% of patients improve within 3 weeks and 70% eventually recover fully (may take 12–18 months).
- Poor prognostic factors: complete palsy/severe pain at onset, age >60 years, no recovery at 3 weeks, associated diabetes/pregnancy.

Eye care

- Ophthalmology referral
- Regular topical lubricants during the day and thicker viscosity at night
- Nocturnal eye taping/eye patch

Surgical options – can be discussed on an outpatient basis if no resolution with medical treatment

- Facial nerve decompression – in trauma settings
- Facial reanimation – pulls the face up to a more symmetrical position
  - Static (non-movement) – fascia lata sling
  - Dynamic (can allow some movement) – digastric muscle transfer, temporalis muscle, hypoglossal-facial anastomosis
- Oculoplastic surgery – blepharoplasty, eyelid loading, lateral/medial canthopexy, brow lift

---

RISKS OF ORAL CORTICOSTEROIDS

- Gastrointestinal – nausea, vomiting, reflux, ulcer, change in appetite, weight gain
- Musculoskeletal – muscle weakness, osteoporosis, avascular necrosis of femoral head
- Visual – blurred vision
- Mood – nervousness, restlessness, difficulty sleeping, altered mood
- Immunosuppression
- Swollen face
- Easy bruising
- Hyperglycaemia and worsening of diabetic control if diabetic
- High blood pressure

Discharge and follow-up

- Patients with Bell's palsy do not routinely need to be admitted
- Follow-up in emergency clinic/otology/facial nerve clinic after 4–6 weeks to assess for resolution
- Patients with a non-Bell's palsy cause should be treated and followed-up accordingly

RED FLAGS

- Inability to close eye
- Signs and symptoms of central causes

WHEN TO REFER FROM PRIMARY CARE

- Most patients with Bell's palsy can be commenced on corticosteroids in primary care and referred to emergency clinic for review in 4–6 weeks if
  - No improvement
  - Diagnostic uncertainty
  - Re-innervation symptoms (e.g. gustatory sweating)

Rhinology

Chapter 24

Rhinosinusitis

Background

Rhinosinusitis can be acute (with symptoms lasting less than 12 weeks) or chronic (more than 12 weeks). In adults, inflammation of the nose and paranasal sinuses results in nasal obstruction or discharge, and at least one of either facial pain, hyposmia or endoscopic/radiological signs of inflammation. This is similar in children; however, cough replaces a change in smell. Acute rhinosinusitis (ARS) is often a consequence of the common cold; symptoms typically last for less than 10 days. This can generally be managed with supportive measures in the community. The most common causative organisms are respiratory viruses and, therefore, antibiotics are rarely useful. A small proportion of patients with ARS will develop acute bacterial rhinosinusitis. Patients will generally experience discoloured nasal discharge, facial pain, pyrexia, and/or elevated inflammatory markers. It is important to be able to recognise the uncommon but life-threatening complications of ARS (Table 24.1). Chronic rhinosinusitis (CRS) is common and can have a long-term impact on the quality of life. It has a complex multifactorial aetiology related to interaction between the sinus respiratory epithelium and external irritants (including microorganisms, allergens, pollutants and tobacco smoke). CRS is subdivided into primary or secondary forms, both of which have varying phenotypes (Table 24.2). Patients with rhinosinusitis often have a fluctuating clinical course, sometimes requiring conservative management, escalating through medical therapy options and even surgery. In some refractory cases, patients have persistent symptoms despite maximal medical therapy and surgery.

History

Symptoms

- Onset, timing and duration
- Frequency of blockage/discharge/facial pain
- Better or worse
- Laterality especially distinguishing between unilateral and bilateral symptoms
- Exacerbating or relieving factors
- Previous episodes including previous treatments and their effects
- Preceding URTI symptoms

DOI: 10.1201/b23238-31

Table 24.1 Complications of acute rhinosinusitis

Classification	Examples
Orbital	Periorbital cellulitis (Chandler's classification – preseptal cellulitis, orbital cellulitis, subperiosteal abscess, orbital abscess)
Intracranial	Meningitis, extradural/subdural abscess, cerebral abscess, cavernous sinus thrombosis
Osseous	Osteomyelitis, Pott's puffy tumour (frontal osteomyelitis with subperiosteal abscess)

Systems

- Nasal/sinus – blockage, obstruction, congestion, discharge, postnasal drip, facial pain, facial pressure, reduced sense of smell, anosmia, cacosmia, epistaxis
- Visual – change in vision (blurring, double vision, reduced colour vision), pain on eye movement, photophobia
- Intracranial – nausea, vomiting, headache, loss of consciousness, seizures, rashes, features of meningism, swinging pyrexia

Past medical history

- Previous sinus surgery
- History of atopy (asthma, eczema, hayfever)
- Adult-onset asthma – associated with Type 2 eosinophilic CRS
- Long-term conditions, especially primary ciliary dyskinesia, cystic fibrosis, granulomatosis with polyangiitis, eosinophilic granulomatosis with polyangiitis

Social history

- Smoking, occupational exposure to dust/irritants
- Exposure to animals/pets
- Performance status (if considering surgery)
- Impact of symptoms on quality of life and activities of daily living (VAS and SNOT-22 scoring systems)

Table 24.2 Classifications of primary and secondary CRS

CRS type	Localisation	Examples of phenotypes
Primary	Unilateral	Isolated sinusitis, allergic fungal rhinosinusitis
	Bilateral	Type 2 eosinophilic CRS (often with nasal polyps), non-type 2 CRS
Secondary	Unilateral	Odontogenic, fungal ball, sinonasal tumour
	Bilateral	Mechanical – primary ciliary dyskinesia, cystic fibrosis Autoimmune – granulomatosis with polyangiitis, eosinophilic granulomatosis with polyangiitis (Churg-Strauss) Immune – immunodeficiency

Examination

If there are concerns regarding serious complications of ARS, then a detailed examination of the visual and neurological systems should be undertaken as detailed next. Otherwise, patients with rhinosinusitis warrant examination of the nose to assess for objective signs of mucosal disease.

- General inspection – nasal collapse on inspiration, overt nasal discharge
- Nose – assess for objective signs of inflammation/disease with anterior rhinoscopy or flexible nasoendoscopy (FNE)
  - Nasal polyps
  - Mucopurulent discharge (usually from middle meatus)
  - Oedema/mucosal obstruction
  - Unilateral sinonasal or post nasal space (PNS) mass
- Eye – general inspection, lid oedema, cellulitis, ability to open, proptosis/chemosis
  - Vision – current vision compared to baseline (no change, blurring, colour, shadow, movement)
  - Cranial nerves
    - II (optic) – fields, acuity, relative afferent pupillary defect (RAPD), colour, pupillary reflexes
    - III (oculomotor), IV (trochlear), VI (abducens) – diplopia, ophthalmoplegia, eye movement
- Neurological – GCS, gait, assess for signs of meningism (nuchal rigidity, non-blanching rash, Kernig's sign, Brudzinski's sign)
- Full set of observations – assess for signs of sepsis (fever, tachycardia, hypotension, tachypnoea)

Management

The principle of management for patients with rhinosinusitis is symptom control. Patients can present with a wide spectrum of disease states and management is tailored accordingly. ARS is usually viral and self-limiting. Suspected complications of ARS are usually managed as an inpatient. CRS is initially managed with allergen avoidance, steam inhalations/saline nasal douching and appropriate medical therapy. If this approach fails to achieve symptom control, surgical treatment may be considered.

Investigations

- Nasal pus swab for severe/complex ARS
- Blood tests – FBC and eosinophil count, U&E, ESR, CRP, total IgE
  - Consider autoimmune screen if suspecting vasculitic CRS
  - Allergy testing if strong history of atopy (skin prick testing or RAST)

Imaging

- CT sinus (Figure 24.1)
  - Diagnosis – mucosal changes within sinuses and/or ostiomeatal complex
  - Operative planning – assess extent of disease and to identify key anatomical landmarks (cribriform plate, lamina papyracea, anterior ethmoidal artery and additional sinus cells – Haller, Agger Nasi and Onodi cells)

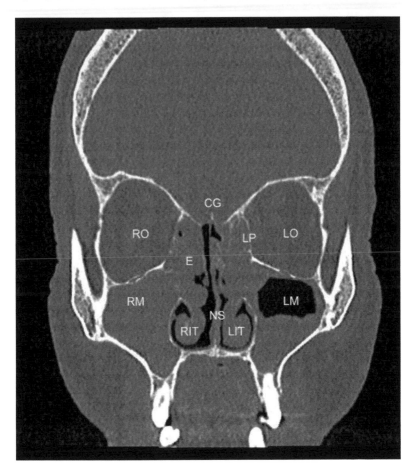

Figure 24.1 Coronal CT sinuses demonstrating bilateral sinonasal polyposis and mucosal thickening and opacification of the maxillary antra and ethmoid air cells. There is complete opacification of the ostiomeatal units. (*Abbreviations:* CG: crista galli, E : ethmoid air cells, LIT: left inferior turbinate, LM : left maxillary sinus, LO: left orbit, LP: lamina papyracea, NS: nasal septum, RIT: right inferior turbinate, RM: right maxillary sinus, RO: right orbit.)

Conservative – symptomatic relief for viral ARS

- Nasal decongestant <10 days + steam inhalations
- Saline nasal douching
- Simple analgesia

Medical – management commenced in primary care (without the need for routine bloods and imaging)

- Intranasal or oral corticosteroids
- Nasal decongestant <10 days + steam inhalations
- Saline nasal douching

- Antibiotics (not first line treatment)
  - In patients with signs/symptoms suggesting acute bacterial rhinosinusitis (amoxicillin, clarithromycin are commonly used)
  - Immunomodulation in CRS (macrolides)

Surgical – to improve sinus ventilation, mucociliary clearance and future application of topical therapy in patients who are refractory to maximal medical therapy

- Functional endoscopic sinus surgery (FESS)
  - Limited FESS – depending on which sinuses are involved
  - 'Full house' FESS – typically involves opening all sinuses (anterior and posterior ethmoidectomy, middle meatal antrostomy bilaterally, sphenoidotomy and frontal sinus opening)
  - Extended FESS – extensive opening of frontal sinus

Biologics

- Monoclonal antibody (Dupilumab) is currently approved only for severe CRS with nasal polyps.

RED FLAGS

- Orbital – periorbital oedema/erythema, globe displacement, ophthalmoplegia, double vision, reduced visual acuity
- Intracranial – severe headache, signs of meningitis, neurological signs
- Osseous – frontal swelling/cellulitis
- Nasal – unilateral symptoms (bleeding, crusting), cacosmia
- Systemic – signs of sepsis

WHEN TO REFER FROM PRIMARY CARE

To ED
- Red flags suggesting complications of ARS (orbital, intracranial, osseous)

To rhinology clinic
- ARS: More than 2 episodes per year or after no improvement with oral antibiotics
- CRS: Residual significant symptoms after 6–12 weeks of medical therapy
- Presence of systemic disease (vasculitis or immune disorder) suggesting secondary diffuse CRS

COMPLICATIONS OF FESS

- Nasal – altered smell, epistaxis
- Orbital – epiphora by damage to nasolacrimal apparatus, damage to extraocular eye muscles, orbital haematoma, loss of vision
- Intracranial – CSF leak, meningitis

Chapter 25

Anosmia

Background

Anosmia is a sensory deficit characterised by complete loss of smell, as opposed to other smell disturbances such as hyposmia (reduced sense of smell). It is often associated with a perceived disturbance in taste, as gustation relies significantly on the sense of smell. Causes for smell disturbance and anosmia can be broadly divided into two groups: conductive or sensorineural, and these can be temporary or permanent. The most common cause of anosmia is following a viral upper respiratory infection; this has seen an increased prevalence during the COVID-19 pandemic. The next most common cause is inflammatory sinonasal disease (chronic rhinosinusitis) with or without nasal polyposis. Table 25.1 outlines the main causes of olfactory dysfunction. Anosmia can have significant quality of life implications, depending on hobbies and occupations that rely on smell and taste (e.g. those working in the food and beverage industry). A detailed history and examination are key in diagnosis and guiding management.

History

Symptoms

- Onset, timing and duration
- Fluctuating nature, e.g. anosmia versus hyposmia
- Better or worse
- Exacerbating or relieving factors
- Preceding upper respiratory tract infection (URTI) symptoms
- Previous episodes including previous treatments and their effects
- Trauma history

Systems

- Nasal/sinus – blockage, obstruction, congestion, discharge, postnasal drip, facial pain, facial pressure, reduced sense of smell, anosmia, cacosmia, epistaxis
- Visual – change in vision, pain on eye movement, photophobia
- Neurological – headaches, syncope, seizures, loss of consciousness, vomiting

Past medical history

- Previous nasal/sinus surgery
- Chronic rhinosinusitis

DOI: 10.1201/b23238-32

Table 25.1 Causes of olfactory dysfunction

Conductive	Rhinosinusitis, polyps, foreign body, tumours
Infective	Post-viral (URTI, COVID-19)
Neurological	Alzheimer's disease, Parkinson's disease, epilepsy, multiple sclerosis, olfactory neuroblastoma
Metabolic/endocrine	Diabetes mellitus, hypothyroidism, hypogonadism, hypoadrenalism, chronic renal/liver failure, vitamin/mineral deficiency
Vasculitis	Sarcoidosis, granulomatosis with polyangiitis
Trauma	Head, nose, skull base
Congenital	Kallman syndrome, primary congenital anosmia
Iatrogenic	Sinonasal or neurosurgery, skull base radiotherapy
Drugs	Cocaine, nifedipine, diltiazem, methotrexate, amitriptyline
Other	Idiopathic, age

- Post-viral syndromes – e.g. long COVID-19
- Neurological disorders – Parkinson's disease, Kallman syndrome

Social history

- Smoking, alcohol status
- Performance status
- Impact on quality of life, activities of daily living and hobbies

Examination

- General inspection – nasal deformity/collapse
- Anterior rhinoscopy – nasal polyps, foreign body or other obstruction
- Flexible nasoendoscopy (FNE) – mass lesion, nasal polyps, features of chronic rhinosinusitis
- Cranial nerve examination

Management

The principle of management in patients with anosmia is to find an underlying cause (if any) which can then be treated. This can often address their anosmia. In other cases, smell retraining can help the patient cope with their loss of smell.

Investigations

- Formal smell grading can be useful to quantify true anosmia (usually only used in tertiary smell clinics/research centres)
  - University of Pennsylvania Smell Identification Test (UPSIT)
  - Brief Smell Identification Test (BSIT)
  - Connecticut Chemosensory Clinical Research Centre orthonasal olfactory test (CCRCT)

- Blood tests (used in select cases)
  - FBC, U&Es, LFT – screen for underlying disease
  - Vitamin and mineral screen (including vitamin A, B1, B6, B12, calcium, folate, iron, zinc, magnesium, calcium) – if suspecting deficiency
  - Endocrine screen – TFT, HbA1c, cortisol, FSH, LH, oestrodiol, serum testosterone, prolactin – hypothyroidism, diabetes, Cushing's disease, hypogonadism
  - Vasculitis screen

Imaging

- CT sinuses – if chronic rhinosinusitis and planning surgery
- MRI skull base – if negative FNE and unclear aetiology to exclude olfactory cleft lesions (e.g. olfactory neuroblastoma, meningioma)

Conservative

- Smell retraining
- Support groups – e.g. Fifth Sense charity
- Health and safety guidance – e.g. checking food expiry dates and smoke alarms

Medical

- Oral corticosteroid (1 mg/kg, max 60 mg prednisolone) once a day can be trialled (especially if post-viral).
- Appropriate medical treatment of underlying inflammatory sinonasal disease or other cause (e.g. endocrine disorder).
- Supplements (in deficiency).
  - Omega-3 – protective against olfactory loss during post-viral recovery
  - Zinc
  - Intranasal vitamin A

Surgical

- Limited role unless evidence of chronic rhinosinusitis with polyps
- Neoplastic disease can be managed with surgery but often with no improvement in sense of smell post-operatively

Discharge and follow-up

- Patients are usually managed on an outpatient basis and can be followed-up depending on the cause.

RED FLAGS

- Epistaxis (unilateral)
- Nasal unilateral symptoms (crusting, obstruction)
- Cacosmia
- Headaches
- Visual symptoms

WHEN TO REFER FROM PRIMARY CARE

Rhinology clinic via cancer referral pathway

- Any red flags as mentioned above

Routine rhinology clinic

- No improvement in symptoms after 12 weeks

Head and neck

Chapter 26

Head and neck malignancy

Background

For the ENT surgeon, head and neck malignancy usually encompasses tumours of the nasopharynx, oropharynx, hypopharynx, larynx and thyroid. For the purposes of this chapter, we will focus on the most commonly involved anatomical sites: oropharyngeal, hypopharyngeal and laryngeal malignancies. Traditional risk factors of such tumours are well established and include smoking, alcohol and low socio-economic status. There is also a strong association between human papilloma virus (HPV) (especially subtypes 16 and 18) and oropharyngeal cancer. HPV-positive tumours tend to have a better prognosis and are more radiosensitive. Table 26.1 summarises the anatomical structures associated with each cancer site. Patients can present in a variety of ways that can overlap depending on tumour site. Management generally involves histopathological confirmation of the diagnosis (biopsy) and subsequent treatment governed by patient and tumour factors in an MDT approach. Treatment modalities include radiotherapy, chemotherapy, surgery and palliation.

History

Symptoms – can be variable

- Onset, timing and duration
- Better or worse
- Laterality (if neck lump/pain)
- Exacerbating or relieving factors

Systems

- Airway – difficulty in breathing, SOB, aspiration/choking, drooling
- Oesophagus – dysphagia, odynophagia, regurgitation
- Voice – change in voice
- Systemic features – unexplained persistent fever, weight loss, malnutrition, night sweats, reduced appetite

Past medical history

- Immunocompromise (especially HIV)
- Previous malignancy and treatment (especially radiotherapy)

DOI: 10.1201/b23238-34

Table 26.1 Anatomical structures associated with oropharyngeal, hypopharyngeal and laryngeal malignancy

Cancer site	Anatomical structures
Oropharynx	Palatine tonsils, soft palate, tongue base, lingual tonsil, vallecula, lingual surface of epiglottis, posterior pharyngeal wall (anterior to C2 and C3)
Hypopharynx	Piriform fossae, posterior pharyngeal wall (inferior to C3), post-cricoid
Larynx	Supraglottis (epiglottis, aryepiglottic folds, false cords, arytenoids), glottis (vocal cords), subglottis

VARIABLE PRESENTING SYMPTOMS OF HEAD AND NECK MALIGNANCY

- Dysphonia
- Disorders of swallow (dysphagia, odynophagia)
- Unexplained lymphadenopathy
- Unilateral otalgia
- Chronic cough
- Sore throat >3 weeks
- Obstructive symptoms – stridor, respiratory distress
- Constitutional symptoms – unexplained persistent fever, weight loss, malnutrition, night sweats, reduced appetite

Social history

- Smoking, alcohol status
- Nutritional status
- Performance status
- Impact on quality of life, activities of daily living and hobbies (e.g. singing)

Examination

- General inspection – unkempt, malnourished
- Oral cavity – assess dentition, oral lesions
- Oropharynx – asymmetric tonsillar enlargement, tongue base assessment, palpation
- Neck – range of motion, palpation for lymphadenopathy
- Voice – speaking in full sentences, quality of voice, hoarseness
- Signs of respiratory distress and stridor
- Flexible nasoendoscopy (FNE) – systematic assessment of tongue base, posterior pharyngeal wall, vallecula, epiglottis, piriform fossae and vocal cords
  - Assess for lesions – tumours can be ulcerated and exophytic
  - Pooling of blood or saliva in vallecula may indicate hidden hypopharyngeal tumour
  - Vocal cord mobility/fixation
  - Assess the residual airway

Management

The principle of management for patients with head and neck malignancy is a shared management plan taking into account patient wishes. There is a wide spectrum of treatment options, ranging from palliation to radical surgery. This is often dependent on tumour and patient factors and, therefore, an MDT approach must be taken for all patients. Imaging may need to be performed before biopsy, as this can disrupt radiological assessment of tumour stage. Careful discussion and counselling of patients is essential as primary (chemo)radiotherapy and/or surgical resection may result in significant changes in the patient's quality of life. Palliative treatment may be utilised in patients presenting with advanced tumours, in those where extensive comorbidities preclude active management, or in cases of patient choice.

Bedside investigations

- Blood tests – not routinely required in a clinic setting but can be employed for a baseline status

Imaging

- CT neck and thorax with contrast to assess (Figure 26.1):
  - Radiological staging of primary site (Table 26.2)
  - Cervical lymph node involvement
  - Metastatic disease (commonly lung)
- Ultrasound neck + fine needle aspiration cytology (FNAC)/core biopsy – cervical nodal involvement
- MRI neck and thorax – for more detailed assessment of involvement in thyroid cartilage or tongue base if unclear on CT
- PET-CT
  - If other cross-sectional imaging identified no primary
  - To assess for distant metastasis/other malignancies
  - After non-surgical treatment to assess for residual disease

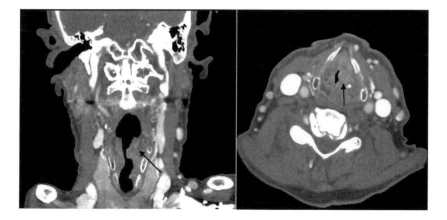

Figure 26.1 Coronal (left) and axial (right) CT images of the neck showing an ulcerating left transglottic tumour (black arrows) involving the left aryepiglottic fold and true vocal cord. There is extension to the anterior commissure and probable involvement of the contralateral cord with invasion of the left para glottic fat. The laryngeal cartilages are intact with no evidence of destruction or extra laryngeal spread. Bilateral small laryngoceles are noted. The radiological staging is that of a T3 tumour.

Table 26.2 TNM classification for head and neck malignancies

Stage	Oropharynx	Hypopharynx	Supraglottis	Glottis	Subglottis
T1	<2 cm in greatest dimension	<2 cm and one subsite	One subsite	a – one vocal cord b – both cords	Subglottis only
T2	2–4 cm in greatest dimension	2–4 cm or more than one subsite or adjacent site	More than one adjacent subsite or outside supraglottis	Extending to supraglottis or impaired vocal cord movement	Extends to vocal cords with normal/impaired mobility
T3	>4 cm in greatest dimension	>4 cm or fixation of hemilarynx	Limited to larynx with vocal cord fixation		
T4a T4b	Moderately advanced local disease Very advanced local disease	Through thyroid cartilage/beyond larynx Prevertebral space, mediastinum or encases carotid			

Histological diagnosis

- Confirm suspected head and neck malignancy – biopsy (usually under general anaesthetic)
  - Panendoscopy + biopsy – suspected oropharyngeal/hypopharyngeal lesions
  - Microlaryngoscopy + biopsy – suspected laryngeal lesions

Early tumours (typically T1/T2)

- Oropharynx
  - Surgery – open, transoral laser microsurgery (TLM) or transoral robotic surgery (TORS)
  - Radiotherapy
  - Neck treatment – neck dissection or radiotherapy
- Hypopharynx
  - Radiotherapy
- Larynx
  - Surgery – TLM or TORS for supraglottic tumours
  - Radiotherapy

Advanced tumours (typically T3/T4)

- Oropharynx
  - Chemoradiotherapy
  - Surgery – primary resection +/– flap
  - Neck treatment – neck dissection or radiotherapy
  - Palliation
- Hypopharynx
  - Chemoradiotherapy

- Surgery (T4/recurrence) – total laryngopharyngectomy with pharyngeal reconstruction
  - Partial pharyngectomy – patch repair with radial forearm free flap, anterolateral thigh-free flap or pectoralis major pedicled flap
  - Total pharyngectomy – circumferential reconstruction with jejunal free flap/anterolateral thigh free flap or gastric transposition pedicled flap
  - Consider postoperative radiotherapy
- Neck treatment – radiotherapy or surgery (selective or modified radical neck dissection dependent on nodal status)
- Palliation
- Larynx
  - Chemoradiotherapy
  - Surgery – total laryngectomy preferred if tumour invasion through cartilage
  - Neck treatment – chemoradiotherapy or surgery (selective or modified radical neck dissection dependent on nodal status) and consider postoperative chemoradiotherapy
  - Palliation

Recurrent disease

- Salvage surgery
- Radical radiotherapy can only be delivered once to each anatomical area
- Palliation

Postoperative hospital stay (surgical resection)

- Prolonged – typically 2–4 weeks
- Laryngectomy – no patent upper airway, airflow through laryngectomy stoma only (neck breather)
- NBM for 1–2 weeks – tube feeding until contrast swallow excludes leak
- Laryngectomy stoma/tracheostomy training – patient and family
- Swallowing and voice rehabilitation can continue for many months postoperatively. Voice options include:
  - Tracheo-oesophageal puncture
  - Oesophageal speech
  - Electrolarynx

Discharge and follow-up

- Patients with head and neck malignancy are usually followed-up lifelong to monitor for signs of recurrence and any other health-related problems.
- This typically follows:
  - 1–2 years – every 4–6 weeks
  - 3–5 years – every 3–6 months
  - >5 years – yearly

POOR PROGNOSTIC FEATURES

- Patient factors – advanced age, multiple comorbidities, alcohol, smoking
- Histological factors – HPV negative, poorly differentiated tumours
- Tumour factors – advanced disease and metastases, hypopharyngeal site

MEMBERS OF THE MDT CLOSELY INVOLVED IN THE MANAGEMENT OF HEAD AND NECK MALIGNANCY

- Otolaryngology
- Maxillofacial and plastic surgery
- Oncology
- Palliative care team
- Anaesthetics
- Radiology
- Histopathology
- Dietician
- Speech and language therapy
- Head and neck cancer nurse specialist
- Physiotherapist and occupational therapy
- Community support teams – GP, Macmillan cancer support, district nurses, psychologist

ADVERSE EFFECTS OF RADIOTHERAPY

- Pain
- Skin erythema
- Mucositis
- Fibrosis and scarring of pharynx and larynx
- Dysphagia
- Lymphoedema
- Stiffness of jaw, neck and shoulders

COMPLICATIONS OF LARYNGECTOMY

- Wound infection/seroma/dehiscence
- Skin necrosis
- Pharyngocutaneous fistula – may require tube feeding or further reconstructive surgery
- Hypocalcaemia and hypothyroidism
- Pharyngeal stenosis and dysphagia
- Tongue weakness (damage to hypoglossal nerve)
- Stoma stenosis
- Carotid artery blowout

WHEN TO REFER FROM PRIMARY CARE

- Unexplained neck lump persisting >3 weeks
- Unexplained hoarse voice >3 weeks and age >45 years
- Unexplained sore throat >3 weeks

Chapter 27

Malignancy of unknown primary

Background

Head and neck malignancy of unknown primary pertains to a diagnosis of metastatic cancer in lymph nodes of the neck with no obvious primary site. Patients usually present with an isolated enlarged neck node. The majority of unknown primary metastasis originate from occult oropharyngeal primaries which become apparent only on PET imaging or histological assessment following diagnostic tonsillectomy or tongue base mucosectomy. It is important to identify the potential primary site, if possible, to limit the field of irradiation, avoiding unnecessary side effects. The assessment and work-up of such presentations are done in a MDT setting.

History

Symptoms

- Onset, timing and duration
- Laterality
- Progression
- Exacerbating or relieving factors

Systems

- Airway – difficulty in breathing, SOB, aspiration/choking
- Oesophagus – dysphagia, odynophagia, regurgitation
- Voice – change in voice
- Nose – obstruction, unilateral discharge, change in smell, cacosmia, epistaxis, facial pain (nasopharyngeal tumour)
- Ear – unilateral hearing loss (secondary to otitis media with effusion [OME] in nasopharyngeal tumour)
- Systemic features – unexplained persistent fever, weight loss, malnutrition, night sweats, reduced appetite

Past medical history

- Immunocompromise (especially HIV)
- Previous malignancy and treatment (radiotherapy)

DOI: 10.1201/b23238-35

Social history

- Smoking, alcohol status
- Nutritional status
- Performance status
- Impact on quality of life, activities of daily living and hobbies

Examination

- General inspection – unkempt, malnourished
- Neck lump – location, size, solitary/multiple, overlying skin changes, consistency, tethering
- Neck – range of motion and torticollis
- Oral cavity – assess dentition, oral lesions
- Oropharynx – asymmetric tonsillar enlargement, tongue base (palpate)
- Voice – speaking in full sentences, quality of voice, hoarseness
- Signs of respiratory distress and stridor
- FNE – systematic assessment of postnasal space, posterior pharyngeal wall, tongue base, vallecula, laryngeal inlet, piriform fossae
  - Assess for lesions – tumours can be ulcerated/exophytic or submucosal.
  - Pooling of blood or saliva in vallecula may indicate hidden hypopharyngeal tumour.
  - Vocal cord mobility/fixation.
  - Assess the residual airway.

Management

The principle of management in patients with malignancy of unknown primary is early recognition and identification of the primary site. This allows targeted treatment following multidisciplinary team (MDT) discussion considering tumour factors, patient factors and patient choice.

Bedside

- Bloods – baseline health measure – FBC, U&Es

Imaging

- Core biopsy (freehand or US-guided)
  - Advantage of core biopsy over fine needle aspiration is human papillomavirus (HPV) identification.
  - HPV positivity usually implies an oropharyngeal primary.
  - MRI neck – better than CT at assessment of the oropharynx soft tissues (e.g. primary tonsil tumours)
  - CT neck and thorax with contrast to assess:
    - Radiological staging of primary site
    - Cervical lymph node involvement
    - Metastatic disease (most commonly lung)
  - PET-CT
    - If other cross-sectional imaging identified no primary
    - To assess for distant metastasis/other malignancies
    - After non-surgical treatment to assess for residual disease

Histological diagnosis – assuming all clinical examination and imaging (+/− PET-CT) is negative, the patient is classified as having a malignancy of unknown primary

Further management involves obtaining a histological diagnosis

- Panendoscopy, tonsillectomy, tongue base mucosectomy.
- Transoral robotic (TORS) tongue base mucosectomy is preferred with blind tongue base biopsies becoming less utilised.

Conservative management/palliation

- Palliative radiotherapy in those unfit for surgical treatment or advanced disease

Radical treatment – surgery/chemoradiotherapy

- Primary surgery is dependent on the primary site – usually TORS oropharyngectomy (Figure 27.1).
- Small volume nodal disease – surgery with neck dissection.
- Bulky volume nodal disease or extracapsular spread – dual modality treatment (surgery and radiotherapy and consider chemotherapy).

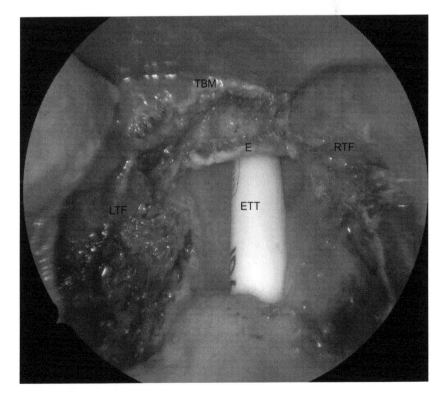

Figure 27.1 Endoscopic image following a tongue base mucosectomy using transoral robotic surgery (TORS). (*Abbreviations:* E: epiglottis, ETT: endotracheal tube, LTF: left tonsil fossa, RTF: right tonsil fossa, TBM: tongue base mucosectomy site.)

WHEN TO REFER FROM PRIMARY CARE

- Unexplained neck lump persisting >3 weeks
- Unexplained hoarse voice >3 weeks and age >45 years
- Unexplained sore throat >3 weeks

ADVERSE EFFECTS OF RADIOTHERAPY

- Pain
- Skin erythema
- Mucositis
- Fibrosis and scarring of pharynx and larynx
- Dysphagia
- Lymphoedema
- Stiffness of jaw, neck and shoulders

Dysphonia

Background

Dysphonia refers to an abnormality of voice, often described as hoarseness. Patients may develop dysphonia due to a number of reasons, ranging from idiopathic cord paralysis, iatrogenic injury, vocal cord lesions (benign and malignant) and neurological disorders (Table 28.1). Patients with persistent, progressive dysphonia over several weeks (especially with risk factors such as smoking, odynophagia and dysphagia) must have an underlying malignancy excluded.

History

Symptoms

- Onset, timing and duration
- Character (e.g. hoarse, quiet, change in pitch, inability to sing/shout)
- Severity – partial or total dysphonia
- Better or worse
- Exacerbating or relieving factors

Systems

- Airway – difficulty in breathing, airway noise, aspiration/choking
- Oesophagus – dysphagia, odynophagia, regurgitation
- Referred otalgia
- Systemic features – unexplained persistent fever, weight loss, malnutrition, night sweats, reduced appetite

Past medical history

- Previous trauma – blunt/penetrating neck, intubation, smoke inhalation
- Recent surgery (affecting course of vagus or recurrent laryngeal nerves) – neck, chest, spinal
- GORD
- Systemic or neurological conditions as listed in Table 28.1

Social history

- Smoking, alcohol status
- Occupation – history of voice use (e.g. teachers, singers, preachers)

DOI: 10.1201/b23238-36

Table 28.1 Causes of dysphonia

Inflammatory	Allergy
	Irritants (e.g. smoke inhalation, alcohol, tobacco)
	LPR or GORD
	Vocal abuse (e.g. regular shouting/singing)
Trauma	Blunt or penetrating laryngeal injury, airway burn, iatrogenic (e.g. intubation)
Infection	Laryngitis (bacterial, viral or fungal)
Malignancy	Dysplasia, laryngeal/hypopharyngeal SCC
Structural	Benign vocal cord lesions (e.g. granuloma, nodule, cyst, Reinke's oedema)
	Laryngeal papillomatosis
	Age-related atrophy
Neuromuscular	Muscle tension dysphonia
	Laryngeal dystonia
	Nerve injury (vagus, recurrent laryngeal)
Neurological	Multiple sclerosis, Parkinson's disease, stroke, myaesthenia gravis
Systemic	Acromegaly, amyloidosis, lupus, sarcoid, hypothyroidism

Abbreviations: LPR, laryngopharyngeal reflux; GORD, gastro-oesophageal reflux; SCC, squamous cell carcinoma.

- Performance status
- Impact on quality of life, activities of daily living and hobbies (e.g. singing)

Examination

- Assessment of voice quality
  - Voice Handicap Index (VHI-10) – subjective rating by patients
  - GRBAS score (global score, roughness, breathiness, asthenia, strain) – clinician score
- Examination of oral cavity
- FNE
  - Vocal cords – structural lesions, phonic gap, vocal cord immobility, muscle tension dysphonia, atrophy
  - Laryngeal inlet – malignancy, signs of LPR/GORD, infection (e.g. candida)
- Complete head and neck examination (cervical lymphadenopathy/masses)

Management

The principles of management in dysphonic patients involves firstly excluding an underlying malignancy and then treating according to the aetiology. If malignancy is suspected, an urgent microlaryngoscopy and biopsy should be performed (covered in more detail in head and neck malignancy chapter). Thereafter, management is usually best managed in a specialist voice setting with speech and language therapy (SLT) input.

Imaging

- CXR – arranged in primary care to exclude underlying respiratory disease
- CT skull base to diaphragm – assess for lesions along course of recurrent laryngeal nerve

Specialist investigations

- Videolaryngostroboscopy (VLS) or videokymography (VKG) – visualise and assess vocal cord movement and symmetry

Conservative

- SLT rehabilitation – especially in vocal cord palsy and issues related to voice misuse (e.g. vocal cord nodules, vocal cord granuloma)
- Lifestyle changes – hydration, weight loss, voice hygiene measures
- Smoking cessation – especially with Reinke's oedema

Medical

- Anti-reflux medication – LPR
- Intra-lesion antivirals and systemic biologics (Avastin) – severe paediatric cases of laryngeal papillomatous disease

Surgical

- Microlaryngoscopy and biopsy – lesions suspicious of malignancy
- Microlaryngoscopy and excision of lesions (e.g. large vocal cord granuloma, polyp, nodules, or cyst if not responding to conservative/medical interventions)
- Microdebridement of laryngeal papilloma – often require repeat procedures due to high rate of recurrence
- Vocal cord medialisation – in cases of vocal cord palsy
  - Vocal cord injection
    - Long-standing/permanent material – autologous fat, calcium hydroxyapatite, polydimethylsiloxane (PDMS)
    - Temporary material – gelatin, collagen, hyaluronic acid, carboxymethylcellulose
  - Thyroplasty

VOICE HYGIENE MEASURES

- Do not shout if possible (use microphones when loud voice is required)
- Regular steam inhalations
- Avoid alcohol, smoking, caffeine throat lozenges (and spicy/acidic food, dairy in LPR)
- Avoid throat clearing/coughing
- Manage snoring if present (weight loss, mandibular advancement device)
- Vocal warm up before singing/talking extensively

RED FLAGS

- Unexplained hoarseness >3 weeks
- Smoking, alcohol history
- Haemoptysis, SOB, stridor
- Recent neck/laryngeal trauma
- Dysphagia
- Neck lump
- Referred otalgia
- Systemic features – unexplained persistent fever, weight loss, malnutrition, night sweats, reduced appetite

WHEN TO REFER FROM PRIMARY CARE

To ED
- Symptoms/signs of airway obstruction

To head and neck clinic via cancer referral pathway
- Unexplained hoarse voice >3 weeks and age >45 years

Routine head and neck clinic
- Absence of red flags (e.g. failed conservative management)

Chapter 29

Thyroid lump

Background

The thyroid gland is an endocrine organ responsible for the production of triiodothyronine (T3), tetraiodothyronine (T4) and calcitonin. Follicular cell-produced T3 and T4 increase metabolism, sensitivity to catecholamines and affect growth. The parafollicular C-cells of the thyroid secrete calcitonin, which reduces circulating calcium in the blood. Thyroid disease can lead to overactive (hyperthyroidism) or underactive (hypothyroidism) thyroid hormone states. There are various causes and classifications of such states (Table 29.1). These conditions are usually managed medically in primary care or by endocrinology, with thyroid blocking or replacing drugs.

This chapter will cover the management of thyroid lumps/masses, which are usually managed by ENT surgeons. Thyroid enlargement can present as a discrete mass or diffuse enlargement (goitre). Thyroid masses may be benign or malignant (Table 29.2). Malignant thyroid masses are typically managed with surgery +/− radioactive iodine and usually have excellent survival outcomes. Benign thyroid masses may be non-hormone secreting or hormone secreting. Management of these can be conservative, medical or surgical depending on the underlying cause, progression and related symptoms. Surgery is typically utilised for large multinodular goitres with compressive symptoms or hormone-secreting masses that are refractory to medical therapy.

History

Symptoms

- Onset, timing and duration
- Better or worse
- Exacerbating or relieving factors

Systems

- Airway – difficulty in breathing, SOB, aspiration/choking, drooling
- Oesophagus – dysphagia, odynophagia, regurgitation
- Voice – change in voice
- Hyperthyroid – heat intolerance, weight loss, increased appetite, night sweats, diarrhoea, anxiety, insomnia
- Hypothyroid – cold intolerance, weight gain, reduced appetite, low mood, hair loss, constipation, irregular/absent periods

DOI: 10.1201/b23238-37

Table 29.1 Causes of hyperthyroidism and hypothyroidism

Hyperthyroidism	Hypothyroidism
Grave's disease (autoimmune)	Hashimoto's thyroiditis (autoimmune, may be hyperthyroid in acute phase)
Toxic multinodular goitre	Iodine deficiency
Solitary thyroid nodule (toxic adenoma)	Iatrogenic – radioiodine, neck radiotherapy, thyroidectomy
De Quervain's viral thyroiditis	Congenital – thyroid agenesis
Drugs – amiodarone, lithium, exogenous iodine	Drugs – amiodarone, contrast media, iodides, lithium, antithyroid medication
	Infiltration – amyloid, sarcoid, haemochromatosis
	Secondary to hypopituitarism (neoplasm, infection, radiotherapy, infiltrative, apoplexy, Sheehan's syndrome – postpartum)
	Tertiary – hypothalamic disorder (neoplasm, trauma)

Past medical history

- Previous radiotherapy or radiation exposure to the head and neck
- Previous neck surgery
- Endocrine disease related to MEN – parathyroid, phaeochromocytoma, marfanoid habitus
- Amyloid, sarcoid, haemochromatosis
- Living/lived in an iodine deprived area
- Family history of thyroid disease/cancer

Table 29.2 Types and characteristics of thyroid masses

Benign	Malignant (thyroid cancer)
Physiological goitre – pregnancy, puberty, idiopathic	Papillary (most common) – typically affects women aged 30–40, tends to spread locally rather than distant metastases
Simple goitre	Follicular – most common in areas of iodine deficiency, typically affects women aged 30–60, tends to spread distantly rather than locally
Multinodular goitre	Hürthle cell – more common in females between 50 and 60, composed of 75–100% Hürthle cells
Endemic goitre – iodine deficiency	Medullary – arises from parafollicular C-cells, associated with MEN type 2 or familial medullary carcinoma
Hyperthyroid goitre	Anaplastic – poorly differentiated, aggressive disease, typically affects women aged 60–80 with patients presenting late (distant metastases) and with a hard-fixed neck mass
Hypothyroid goitre	Thyroid lymphoma – usually non-Hodgkin's type, typically affects women in their 60s as a rapidly growing neck mass

Social history

- Smoking, alcohol status
- Nutritional status
- Performance status
- Impact on quality of life, activities of daily living and hobbies

Examination

- General inspection
  - Hyperthyroidism – fine tremor, palmar erythema, exophthalmos, proptosis
  - Hypothyroidism – overweight, dry coarse skin, puffy face, hands, feet (myxoedema)
- Neck
  - Visible/palpable goitre or nodule (Figure 29.1)
  - Range of motion, palpation for lymphadenopathy

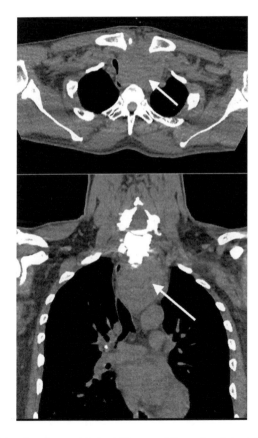

Figure 29.1 Axial (above) and coronal (below) CT scans of the neck and chest demonstrating an enlarged thyroid right-sided goitre with retrosternal extension and significant tracheal compression (white arrows).

- Voice – speaking in full sentences, quality of voice, hoarseness
- Signs of respiratory distress and stridor
- FNE – systematic assessment of tongue base, posterior pharyngeal wall, vallecula, epiglottis, piriform fossae and vocal cords
  - Vocal cord mobility/fixation
  - Assess the residual airway
- Full set of observations – assess for tachy-/bradycardia in hyper and hypothyroid states, respectively

Management

The principle of management for patients presenting with a thyroid mass is confirmation of benign or malignant thyroid enlargement. Patients with uncomplicated hyper- and hypothyroidism are managed medically and onward referral to ENT surgeons is usually indicated only in cases where the disease is refractory to medical therapy. ENT management of thyroid disease is also required in large compressive goitres or cases of suspected/confirmed malignancy. Patients with suspected malignancy are typically worked up in a multidisciplinary setting with imaging, cytology, surgery and radiotherapy/iodine treatment.

Bedside investigations

- Blood tests
  - Thyroid function tests
  - Medullary carcinoma (MTC) – calcitonin, screen for hyperparathyroidism and phaeochromocytoma, genetic screening in proven MTC

Imaging

- US neck +/– FNAC (if indeterminate/suspicious/malignant nodules on USS)
  - Assess position, shape, size, margins, content, echogenicity and vascular pattern of nodules/masses
  - Risk of malignancy on US appearance according to "U" classification (Table 29.3)

Table 29.3 Ultrasound "U" classification of thyroid nodules developed by the British Thyroid Association (BTA)

Classification	Description	Features
U1	Normal	No nodules
U2	Benign	Hyperechoic or isoechoic, cystic changes, peripheral calcification, peripheral vascularity
U3	Indeterminate	Solid, homogenous, marked hyperechoic or hypoechoic, mixed/central vascularity
U4	Suspicious	Solid, hypoechoic, disrupted peripheral calcification, lobulated outline
U5	Malignancy	Solid, hypoechoic, irregular outline, micro/globular calcification, intranodal vascularity, taller than wider, associated lymphadenopathy

Table 29.4 Cytological (FNAC) "Thy" classification of thyroid nodules and onward management developed by the British Thyroid Association (BTA)

Classification	Description	Onward management	Risk of malignancy (%)
Thy1	Insufficient specimen	Repeat FNAC	
Thy2	Benign	Clinical follow up and consider repeat FNAC in 3–6 months	<10
Thy3a	Atypia of unknown significance	Repeat FNAC or diagnostic hemithyroidectomy	5–15
Thy3f	Suspicious of follicular neoplasm	Offer diagnostic hemithyroidectomy	15–30
Thy4	Suspicious of malignancy	Offer diagnostic hemithyroidectomy	60–75
Thy5	Malignant	Discuss at MDT meeting – usually for total thyroidectomy +/– central node clearance	97–100

- Risk of malignancy on cytology according to "Thy" classification (Table 29.4)
    - Very useful in papillary thyroid cancer
    - Less accurate in follicular thyroid cancer (differentiation between benign adenoma and carcinoma is based on peri-vascular or peri-capsular invasion – therefore, usually requires diagnostic hemithyroidectomy)
- CT neck and thorax
    - Staging in malignancy (tumour, node, metastasis staging classification [TNM])
    - Assessment of size and retrosternal extension in goitre (can use MRI neck and chest)

Conservative – watch and wait

- Benign nodule/goitre with no compressive symptoms

Medical (primary care/endocrinology)

- Patients with hyper or hypothyroidism.
- Thyroid stimulating hormone (TSH) suppression with hormone replacement (levothyroxine) can potentially reduce malignancy growth rate.

Surgical (after MDT discussion)

- Hemithyroidectomy – nodules with Thy3a/3f or Thy4 cytology
- Total thyroidectomy +/– central node (level VI) clearance
    - Thy5 cytology
    - Tumours > 4 cm
    - Any size tumour with associated multifocal disease, extrathyroidal spread, familial disease, positive lymph nodes, distant metastases
    - MTC should have total thyroidectomy + level VI neck dissection

- Completion thyroidectomy following diagnostic hemithyroidectomy that confirms malignancy
  - Not required in low-risk unifocal, intrathyroidal lesions <4 cm with clinically/radiologically negative nodes
- Neck dissection – not routinely recommended (risk of recurrent laryngeal nerve/parathyroid damage)
  - Selective neck dissection for confirmed lymph node metastases

Radiotherapy and chemotherapy

- Radiotherapy can help control local symptoms in inoperable disease (usually MTC or anaplastic carcinoma).
- Chemotherapy (tyrosine kinase inhibitors) can help with local symptoms.
- Palliative chemoradiotherapy is usually the mainstay of care in patients with anaplastic carcinoma.

Post-operative management

- Check calcium (+/– PTH levels) within 24 hours and treat hypocalcaemia as required
- Commence levothyroxine (typically between 1.5 and 2 micrograms/kg)
- Check thyroglobulin levels after 6 weeks (to monitor recurrence)
- Consider radioiodine (I^{131}) ablation in high-risk patients (Table 29.5)
- Refer persistent dysphonic patients to SLT
- Refer persistent hypocalcaemia (secondary to hypoparathyroidism) to endocrinology

Discharge and follow-up

- Patients with thyroid cancer are usually closely followed-up in MDT setting.
- Papillary and follicular carcinoma – lifelong follow-up with thyroglobulin +/– calcium monitoring for:
  - Late recurrence
  - Long-term effects of TSH suppression (e.g. atrial fibrillation, osteoporosis)
  - Late effects of radioiodine ablation
- MTC – lifelong follow-up with calcitonin and CEA monitoring

Table 29.5 Risk stratification following thyroid surgery for radioiodine ablation (I^{131})

Radioiodine recommendation	Clinical features
Definite	Tumour >4 cm Any size tumour with extrathyroidal extension Distant metastases
Probable (discuss at MDT)	Unfavourable histology including widely invasive tumour Multiple lymph node involvement, large nodes, extracapsular spread
Not for ablation (meets all criteria)	Tumour <1 cm (unifocal or multifocal) Histology – classical papillary/follicular variant/follicular carcinoma Minimally invasive – no angioinvasion or extrathyroidal spread

COMPLICATIONS OF THYROID SURGERY

- Wound infection/seroma/dehiscence
- Haematoma (see Chapter 16)
- Hypocalcaemia
- Hypothyroidism
- Recurrent laryngeal nerve injury (unilateral – hoarse voice, bilateral – airway obstruction that may require tracheostomy)

RED FLAGS

- Previous head and neck irradiation
- Goitre associated with unexplained hoarseness, stridor or dysphagia
- Painless rapidly enlarging thyroid mass
- Palpable cervical lymphadenopathy
- Children/adolescents with thyroid mass

WHEN TO REFER FROM PRIMARY CARE

To ED

- Airway compromise secondary compression

To head and neck clinic via cancer referral pathway

- Hoarse voice + thyroid goitre
- Children with thyroid mass
- Cervical lymphadenopathy + thyroid goitre
- Rapidly enlarging painless thyroid mass

Chapter 30

Salivary gland mass

Background

There are three sets of major salivary glands (parotid, submandibular and sublingual) and around 600–1,000 minor salivary glands in the submucosa of the head and neck. Saliva has important functions in mechanical cleaning and oral lubrication, antimicrobial activity, digestion and the facilitation of speech, chewing and swallowing. Salivary gland masses commonly occur as a result of inflammatory, neoplastic, infective or obstructive pathologies (Table 30.1). There are a number of other metabolic and less common causes that could account for salivary gland enlargement, but these are outside the context of this chapter. A clear and detailed history will often allow the clinician to differentiate between possible aetiologies.

History

Symptoms

- Onset, timing and duration
- Laterality
- Progression – fluctuating or stable size
- Pain
- Exacerbating or reliving factors (e.g. meals with sialolithiasis)
- Preceding illness (e.g. URTI or other viral illness)
- Associated symptoms – dry mouth, foul taste/purulent discharge, facial pain, facial weakness

Systems

- Airway – difficulty in breathing, SOB, aspiration/choking, drooling
- Swallowing – dysphagia, odynophagia, trismus, oral blood
- Voice – change in voice
- Systemic features/autoimmune – unexplained persistent fever, weight loss, malnutrition, night sweats, reduced appetite, dry eyes, rashes

Past medical history

- History of autoimmune conditions
- Dental history
- Previous head and neck surgery or radiotherapy

DOI: 10.1201/b23238-38

Table 30.1 Causes of salivary gland enlargement

Infective	Bacterial (staphylococcus aureus), viral (coxsackievirus, parainfleunza, influenza, mumps, HIV, parvovirus B19, herpes), TB
Inflammatory	Sjogren's syndrome, granulomatosis with polyangiitis, sarcoidosis
Neoplasm (benign)	Pleomorphic adenoma, Warthin's tumour
Neoplasm (malignant)	Mucoepidermoid carcinoma, adenoid cystic carcinoma, acinic cell carcinoma, malignant transformation pleomorphic adenoma, adenocarcinoma, SCC, lymphoma
Structural	Sialolithiasis (stone), sialectasis (stricture), mucocele

Social history

- Smoking, alcohol status
- Nutritional status
- Performance status
- Impact on quality of life, activities of daily living and hobbies

Examination

- Complete head and neck examination including scalp for skin lesions (cutaneous SCC metastasising to intraparotid lymph nodes)
- Oral cavity (including bimanual palpation) – visible stone at duct orifice, inflammation, discharge, palpate deep parotid lobe
- Inspect gland orifices – floor of the mouth on either side of lingual frenulum (submandibular and sublingual), buccal surface by second upper molar (parotid)
- Salivary gland mass – size (parotid swellings can be anteroinferior to the ear lobe), site, overlying skin changes, mobility, pain
- Neck – range of motion, palpation for lymphadenopathy
- Voice – quality, volume, hoarseness, pitch
- Signs of respiratory distress and stridor
- Cranial nerves (especially facial nerve)
- FNE – systematic assessment of upper aerodigestive tract

Management

The principle of management for patients with salivary gland masses is to distinguish between neoplastic and non-neoplastic causes. Surgical excision is usually the treatment of choice for salivary gland neoplasms, and such cases are usually discussed at the head and neck MDT, taking into account patient and tumour factors. Imaging with US and/or MRI is useful in confirming diagnosis and preoperative planning. Non-neoplastic causes can often be managed medically; autoimmune causes should be discussed with a rheumatologist. Surgical intervention may be appropriate in some cases of stone disease, with options of either minimally invasive (sialendoscopy) techniques for stone removal, or radical surgery with total gland excision.

Bedside tests

- Swab – purulent intraoral discharge (mc&s)
- Blood tests
  - FBC, U&Es, CRP, blood cultures – if suspecting infection/abscess
  - Autoimmune screen, HIV test

Imaging

- US +/– FNAC
  - Best first-line investigation of solid masses
  - Cytology – benign or malignant
  - Can help exclude abscess in acute setting
- MRI (in neoplasm)
  - Detailed assessment of extent of lesion
  - Relationship of mass to local anatomical structures (e.g. facial nerve)
  - Preoperative planning
- CT neck and chest
  - Staging in confirmed malignancy

Treatment options

Sialadenitis (salivary gland inflammation – infective or autoimmune)

- A to E approach as patients may present with airway complications or neck abscess
- Conservative – warm compress, analgesia, hydration, oral hygiene advice
- Medical – antibiotics (oral or IV)
- Rheumatology input if autoimmune cause
- Surgical – parotid abscess can be drained under US guidance

Sialolithiasis (salivary gland stone – more common in submandibular gland)

- Conservative – massage and sialogogues (citrus sweets/fluids that stimulate saliva production)
- Medical – antibiotics (acute infective flare up)
- Surgery
  - Intraoral ductal stone – ductal excision and extraction
  - Sialendoscopy – for small stones <4 mm
  - Submandibular gland excision – larger stones intraglandular or at hilum, recurrent disease

Neoplasm

- Benign
  - Superficial parotidectomy (if deep is lobe not involved)
- Malignant
  - Head and neck MDT
  - Surgical – superficial or total parotidectomy (facial nerve sacrificed if involved) or submandibular gland excision +/– neck dissection
  - Radiotherapy
    - Primary – inoperable tumours for palliation
    - Post-operative (adjuvant) – high-risk tumours (e.g. >4 cm, residual neck disease, adenoid cystic carcinoma)

Discharge and follow-up

- Follow-up is dependent on the underlying diagnosis and patient factors.
- Most cases require long-term follow-up with active surveillance to assess for recurrence that can be even 10–15 years later.

COMPLICATIONS OF PAROTIDECTOMY

- General – infection, bleeding, pain, scar, DVT, PE
- Facial nerve palsy – temporary/permanent
- Salivary fistula
- Haematoma/seroma/sialocele
- Ear lobe numbness (greater auricular nerve palsy/sacrifice)
- Xerostomia
- Frey's syndrome – gustatory sweating due to inappropriate re-innervation of parasympathetic fibres to the skin
- First bite syndrome – pain triggered by salivation on taking first bite of a meal
- Recurrence – even 10–15 years later

RED FLAGS

- Firm, painless mass
- Increasing in size
- Facial nerve weakness
- Paraesthesia/anaesthesia of overlying skin
- Overlying skin changes
- Lump fixation
- Trismus

WHEN TO REFER FROM PRIMARY CARE

To ED

- Sialadenitis with systemic features/sepsis, abscess, deep space neck infection

To head and neck clinic via cancer referral pathway

- Unexplained salivary gland lump in patients >45 years

Chapter 31

Dysphagia

Background

Swallowing difficulties can be due to pathology anywhere between the oral cavity and oesophagus. Dysphagia may occur with either solids and liquids, or both. This may significantly impact a patient's quality of life, leading to dehydration, malnutrition and aspiration. Dysphagia may arise with associated symptoms such as odynophagia (painful swallowing), dysphonia (voice disturbance) and globus sensation (feeling of a lump in the throat). The causes of dysphagia can be divided into acute or chronic (Table 31.1). Management involves confirmation of the diagnosis, exclusion of malignancy and subsequent treatment guided by this. Patients with high dysphagia (localising above the sternal notch) are usually treated in an ENT setting, while low dysphagia is referred to gastroenterology/upper GI surgery. In the acute setting, dysphagia can be associated with imminent airway obstruction, triggering the need for urgent resuscitation and airway management. In an outpatient setting, once obstructive causes are excluded, speech and language therapy (SLT) is often the main focus of treatment for neuromuscular disorders. As always, it is essential that a detailed history is obtained to help guide diagnosis, management and to ultimately enhance patient outcome and quality of life.

History

Symptoms

- Onset, timing and duration
- Severity – partial or total dysphagia
- Type of dysphagia – solid, liquid, both
- Better or worse
- Exacerbating or relieving factors

Systems

- Airway – difficulty in breathing, SOB, aspiration/choking, recurrent chest infections
- Oesophagus – odynophagia, regurgitation, halitosis
- Voice – change in voice
- Referred otalgia
- Systemic features – unexplained persistent fever, weight loss, malnutrition, night sweats, reduced appetite

DOI: 10.1201/b23238-39

Table 31.1 Acute and chronic causes of dysphagia

Acute	
Infection	Tonsillitis, peritonsillar abscess, supraglottitis, deep space neck infection, oral candidiasis
Foreign body ingestion	Food bolus (e.g. meat), foreign object ingestion (e.g. fish bone, battery)
Trauma	Head, blunt/penetrating neck injury, upper aerodigestive tract burns
Neurological	Stroke, lower cranial nerve palsy
Iatrogenic	Post-surgery, chemotherapy, radiotherapy, tracheostomy
Chronic	
Autoimmune	Behcet's syndrome, CREST syndrome/limited scleroderma, dermatomyositis, Sjögren's syndrome, SLE
Congenital	Oesophageal atresia, tracheoesophageal fistula, laryngeal cleft
Head and neck malignancy	Tumours occurring anywhere in the path of swallow – oral, oropharynx, pharyngeal and oesophageal
Inflammatory	Reflux (laryngopharyngeal reflux or gastro-oesophageal reflux), oesophagitis, Plummer-Vinson syndrome
Mechanical	Pharyngeal pouch, stricture, extrinsic compression (thyroid masses)
Motility disorders	Achalasia, hypercontractile oesophagus
Neurological	Multiple sclerosis, myasthenia gravis, motor neurone disease, Parkinson's disease, stroke

Past medical history

- Autoimmune, inflammatory, neuromuscular, or congenital conditions as listed in Table 31.1
- Previous malignancy (resulting in head and neck surgery or chemo/radiotherapy)

Social history

- Smoking, alcohol status
- Nutritional status
- Performance status
- Impact on quality of life, activities of daily living and hobbies

Examination

- General inspection – general appearance (unkempt, malnourished)
- Oral cavity – assess dentition, oral lesions, tongue coating (candida), trismus
- Oropharynx – asymmetric tonsillar enlargement/tongue base (palpate)
- Neck – range of motion, presence of masses/lymphadenopathy
- Voice – quality, volume, hoarseness, pitch
- Stridor/signs of respiratory distress
- FNE – assessment of post-nasal space, posterior pharyngeal wall, tongue base, vallecula, laryngeal inlet, piriform fossae and oesophageal inlet
  - Assess for lesions – tumours may be ulcerated/exophytic or submucosal.

- Vocal cord mobility/fixation.
- Airway assessment.

Management

The principle of management for patients with dysphagia involves a multidisciplinary approach to manage the underlying cause. Diagnostic and management support from neurology, rheumatology, gastroenterology and oral maxillofacial surgery (OMFS) colleagues may be necessary, alongside rehabilitation expertise from SLT and dietitian colleagues.

Bedside tests

- Blood tests – not routinely required
  - FBC (anaemia), U&Es, refeeding bloods, autoimmune screen

Imaging

- CT neck and thorax (with contrast) – assess for malignancy and staging
- Contrast swallow (barium or water soluble)/videofluoroscopy – assess swallow mechanism, presence of pharyngeal pouch/achalasia (Figure 31.1)
- Gastroenterology may employ other tests:
  - OGD to exclude oesophageal malignancy and assess extent and cause of reflux disease, e.g. Barretts oesophagus, hiatus hernia
  - Manometry to assess oesophageal pressure and muscle function, e.g. in achalasia

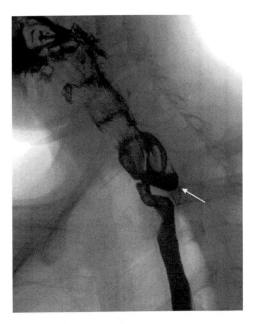

Figure 31.1 Sagittal view of a barium swallow image demonstrating a posterior-sited pharyngeal pouch (white arrow).

Conservative

- Lifestyle changes – sit upright during and after meals, avoid eating 4 hours before bed in reflux.
- Dietary changes, e.g. reducing acidic food/alcohol if there is reflux.
- Smoking cessation.
- SLT rehabilitation/dietitian support.
- Palliative care in malignancy.

Medical

- Calcium channel blockers, Botox injections in motility disorders
- PPI/alginates in reflux disease
- Iron supplementation in Plummer-Vinson syndrome
- Immunosuppressants in autoimmune conditions
- Nutritional support – dietary supplementation/tube feeding (NG tube, gastrostomy)

Surgical

- Oesophageal dilatation
- Pharyngeal pouch – endoscopic division of bar (stapling, CO_2 laser, diathermy, cold steel), cricopharyngeal myotomy, open excision
- Surgical excision of tumour (see head and neck malignancy chapter)

RED FLAGS

- Constitutional symptoms – weight loss, change in appetite, night sweats, unexplained persistent fever
- Progressive dysphagia
- Haemoptysis
- Neck lump
- Voice change
- Referred otalgia
- Previous malignancy
- Airway obstruction – stridor, drooling, respiratory distress

WHEN TO REFER FROM PRIMARY CARE

To ED
- Symptoms of airway obstruction, stroke, foreign body ingestion, sepsis, severe dehydration

To head and neck clinic via cancer referral pathway
- Suspected malignancy (presence of red flags)

Routine head and neck clinic
- Routine referral to ENT in the absence of red flags, e.g. failed conservative management

Paediatrics

Chapter 32

Paediatric hearing loss

Background

Paediatric hearing is a complex subject with many potential causes. Broadly speaking, cases of hearing loss in children can be split into hereditary and acquired forms. In hereditary hearing loss, roughly a third are part of a syndrome and two-thirds non-syndromic. There are more than 400 identified syndromes that result in hearing loss. Table 32.1 summarises some of the most common syndromes. The newborn hearing screening programme (NHSP) was developed to identify children suffering from significant hearing loss in the first few weeks of life and to rehabilitate them early to optimise their speech and language development. In some cases, congenital hearing problems may surface later in childhood (congenital cytomegalovirus [CMV], enlarged vestibular aqueduct) as is the case with acquired causes like otitis media with effusion (OME) (glue ear).

History

Symptoms

- Congenital cases are typically identified early in life through the newborn hearing screening programme (NHSP) (incidence 1–2/1,000 live births).
- Acquired causes can present at any time during childhood.
  - Delayed speech and language development.
  - Reduced hearing noticed by parents/carer/teacher.
  - Behavioural/concentration concerns.
  - History or repeated URTI and AOM.
  - Self-reported hearing loss.

Systems

- Ear – otalgia, otorrhoea, tinnitus, imbalance
- Intracranial – features of meningism
- Change in behaviour – irritability, poor concentration, social isolation, clumsiness
- Systemic features – features of congenital syndrome

Past medical history

- Craniofacial abnormalities or syndromic conditions (risk factor for congenital hearing loss as well as OME)

DOI: 10.1201/b23238-41

Table 32.1 Syndromes associated with hearing loss

Genetic pattern	Syndrome	Hearing loss pattern	Other features
Autosomal dominant	Waardenburg syndrome	Uni/bilateral sensorineural	Pigmentary changes, facial abnormalities
	Branchiootorenal syndrome	Conductive, sensorineural or mixed	Structural ear changes, preauricular cysts, branchial clefts, kidney pathology
	CHARGE syndrome	Conductive, sensorineural or mixed	Coloboma, Heart defect, choanal Atresia, growth Retardation, Genital and Ear abnormalities
	Treacher Collins syndrome	Conductive	Structural facial abnormalities, cleft lip/palate, choanal atresia
	Stickler syndrome	Conductive, sensorineural or mixed	Facial abnormalities, myopia, cataracts, retinal detachment, bone/joint disorders
Autosomal recessive	Usher syndrome	Sensorineural	Retinitis pigmentosa, balance issues
	Pendred syndrome	Sensorineural	Enlarged vestibular aqueduct, goitre
	Jervell and Lange-Nielsen syndrome	Bilateral sensorineural	Long QT arrhythmia
X-linked	Alport syndrome	Sensorineural	Nephritis, myopia, cataracts

- Paediatric primary immune deficiency (e.g. IgA deficiency, Di George syndrome)
- Cystic fibrosis/PCD
- Down's syndrome
- Bacterial meningitis
- Family history of hearing loss (especially in childhood)

Paediatric history

- Antenatal history, complications and risk factors (Box Antenatal history and risk factors)
- Mode of delivery and complications
- Term or pre-term birth
- Neonatal complications including admission to NICU
- Immunisations
- Developmental, growth or behavioural concerns

Social history

- Parental smoking history (risk factor in recurrent AOM/OME)
- Absence of breast feeding (risk factor in recurrent AOM)
- Nursery attendance/multiple siblings (risk factor in recurrent AOM)
- Impact on speech and language/schooling

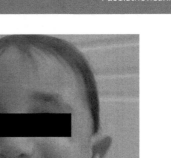

Figure 32.1 Clinical image of a child with Treacher Collins syndrome with characteristic underdevelopment of the zygomatic complex.

Examination

- Assess for functional signs of hearing loss – change in speech clarity, difficulty in hearing conversation in background noise
- General inspection – looking for syndromic features or craniofacial abnormalities (Figure 32.1)
- Ear
  - External examination – aural tags, microtia
  - Otoscopy – OME, congenital abnormalities (e.g. EAC atresia)
- Developmental milestones

Management

The principle of management in patients with paediatric hearing loss is early recognition and management to prevent long-term sequelae such as developmental delay. This involves identification and management of any associated abnormalities, while providing early age-appropriate hearing amplification and rehabilitation. This often requires an MDT approach with close involvement of other allied health professionals such as community paediatrics, clinical genetics, ophthalmology, audiology and support to children/families in the community from the local Teacher of the Deaf (TOD) service.

Hearing tests

- Neonate – electrophysiological tests of hearing through the newborn hearing screening programme (all children born in the UK)
  - Automated otoacoustic emissions test (AOAE)
  - Automated auditory brainstem response test (AABR)
  - All high-risk babies or those failing the above are referred to audiology for further assessment (diagnostic auditory brainstem response test)
- 8 months–3 years – visually reinforced audiometry (VRA)
- 2–5 years – play/performance audiometry
- >5 years – pure tone audiometry (PTA)

Bedside tests

- ECG – Jervell and Lange-Nielsen syndrome

Blood tests

- TORCH infection serology (Box Torch Infections)
- Connexin 26 genetic mutation – most common non-syndromic cause of congenital hearing loss
- Thyroid function – Pendred syndrome
- Additional genetic testing

Imaging

- Renal ultrasound – branchiotorenal syndrome, Alport syndrome
- CT/MRI head

Hearing amplification – dependent on degree of hearing loss and laterality

- Unilateral
  - Some residual hearing and no external ear deformities – conventional air conduction hearing aids
  - External ear deformities (microtia/atresia) – consider bone conduction devices
- Bilateral
  - Some residual hearing and no external ear deformities – conventional hearing aids
  - Bilateral severe/profound hearing loss – consider cochlear implantation

OME

- Conservative management in first 3 months as >50% resolve
- Persistent bilateral hearing loss >25 dB after 3 months – consider use of hearing aids versus insertion of tympanostomy tubes (grommets)

ANTENATAL HISTORY AND RISK FACTORS

- Family history of hearing loss
- Maternal illness – diabetes, fetal alcohol syndrome
- Prematurity or low birth weight
- Severe neonatal jaundice/hyperbilirubinaemia
- Hypoxia or low APGAR score
- Ototoxic medication
- History of TORCH infections
- Admission to neonatal ICU for >48 hours

TORCH INFECTIONS

- Toxoplasmosis
- Other (syphyllis, varicella zoster)
- Rubella
- Cytomegalovirus
- Herpes

Chapter 33

Paediatric sleep disordered breathing

Background

Paediatric sleep disordered breathing is common and can vary from intermittent hypopnea during URTIs to severe obstructive sleep apnoea (OSA). Hypopnea is defined as a 50% reduction in airflow despite respiratory effort, or a >4% desaturation from baseline saturations. Apnoea is a cessation of airflow for greater than 10 seconds. Most children with sleep disordered breathing suffer from the milder end of the spectrum, but it is important to be able to identify and treat higher-risk children to avoid developmental and behavioural sequelae. Children typically become symptomatic around 2 years of age due to growth and development of adenotonsillar tissue. During sleep, reduced upper airway muscle tone and adenotonsillar hypertrophy result in airway obstruction which manifests itself as sleep disordered breathing. For the most part, these patients can be managed in secondary care settings. Higher-risk children (<2 years old, <12 kg, severe cerebral palsy, neuromuscular disorders, significant craniofacial abnormalities, or other significant underlying comorbidities) may need referral to tertiary paediatric units if surgical intervention is required.

History

Symptoms (usually snoring or noisy breathing)

- Onset, timing and duration
- Better or worse
- Exacerbating or relieving factors
- Witnessed apnoeic episodes and frequency (e.g. every night or when child has URTI)
- Child sleeping position (e.g. neck arched backward)
- Cyanotic episodes during sleep
- Frequency of waking up at night
- Nocturnal enuresis
- Daytime somnolence
- Picky eater/avoidance of bulky foods

Systems

- Airway – aspiration/choking episodes, drooling
- Oesophagus – dysphagia, odynophagia

- Voice – change in voice
- Development – failure to thrive, developmental and behavioural issues

Past medical history

- Tonsillitis
- Downs syndrome
- Neuromuscular disorders
- Craniofacial abnormalities
- Sickle cell disease
- Cerebral palsy
- Family history of sleep disordered breathing/OSA

Paediatric history

- Antenatal history and complications
- Mode of delivery and complications
- Term or pre-term birth
- Neonatal complications including admission to NICU
- Immunisations
- Developmental, growth or behavioural concerns

Family history

- Sleep disordered breathing/OSA

Social history

- Parental smoking history
- Impact on quality of life, school, and activities of daily living
- Issues at school – e.g. concentration, poor behaviour, somnolence

Examination

- General inspection – looking for syndromic features or craniofacial abnormalities
- Oropharynx – macroglossia, oropharyngeal crowding, tonsillar hypertrophy (Figure 33.1)
- Craniofacial abnormality, e.g. micrognathia
- Otoscopy – ear examination to exclude coexisting otitis media with effusion

Management

The principle in management for children with sleep disordered breathing is to identify its severity and impact on the child's behaviour and development, tailoring management accordingly. This may be conservative, medical or surgical. When assessing the child in outpatients, if they are fit and well, have a history and examination that is typical of disordered nocturnal breathing and have no risk factors for severe disease, no further investigations are necessary. Many children with mild disease grow out of sleep disordered breathing as their airway diameter increases. In moderate/severe disease, adenotonsillectomy is usually indicated and typically has excellent outcomes. Unlike adults, continuous positive airway pressure (CPAP) is not routinely an option as it is poorly tolerated.

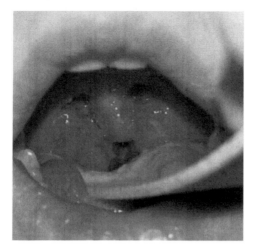

Figure 33.1 Clinical image of enlarged tonsillar tissue in a child.

Investigation

- Polysomnography – gold standard, but not always accessible and is expensive
- Overnight pulse oximetry (high false negative rate)
  - Risk stratifies children based on apnoeas/hypopneas index and nadir SpO_2 (McGill score)

Imaging

- Lateral neck XR – identify postnasal space adenoidal hypertrophy (no longer routinely practiced)

Conservative

- Watch and wait – mild sleep disordered breathing, no developmental or behavioural issues, no risk factors
  - Most sleep disordered breathing is self-limiting, as the child grows and lymphoid tissue regresses.

Medical – shrink adenotonsillar tissue

- Corticosteroid spray/drops
- Leukotrine receptor antagonists (e.g. montelekuast)

Surgical

- Adenotonsillectomy (moderate/severe OSA)

Discharge and follow-up

- Patients with sleep disordered breathing are typically managed on an outpatient basis.
- Children with mild disease may need to be followed-up to ensure there is no symptom progression.

COMPLICATIONS OF ADENOTONSILLECTOMY

- Infection
- Bleeding (including return to theatre) – primary <24 hours, secondary >24 hours
- Pain
- Damage to teeth, lips, gums, tongue, temporomandibular joint
- Velopalatine insufficiency – hypernasal speech, nasal regurgitation

WHEN TO REFER FROM PRIMARY CARE

- History of regular snoring with adenotonsillar hypertrophy
- Symptoms of OSA
- Do not 'watch and wait' in primary care

RISK FACTORS FOR PAEDIATRIC SLEEP DISORDERED BREATHING

- Obesity
- Low birth weight
- Family history
- Downs syndrome
- Craniofacial abnormalities
- Neuromuscular disease
- Cerebral palsy
- Sickle cell disease

Index

Note: Locators in *italics* represent figures and **bold** indicate tables in the text.

Connecticut Chemosensory Clinical Research Centre
orthonasal olfactory test (CCRCT), 126
Continuous positive airway pressure (CPAP), 168
Contralateral routing of sound (CROS) hearing aid, 18
Core biopsy, 138
Corticosteroids, 11, 12, 13, 17, 18, 58, 91, 115, 127
COVID-19 pandemic, 120, 125
CPAP, *see* Continuous positive airway pressure
Cranial nerves, 32, 36, 121
Craniofacial abnormality, 68
Cricothyroid membrane, 50, 50
CROS hearing aid, *see* Contralateral routing of
sound hearing aid
CRS, *see* Chronic rhinosinusitis
CSF leaks, *see* Cerebrospinal fluid leaks
Cyclizine, 104

D

Deep space neck infections, 65–69, **66**
Dix-Hallpike test, 103, 104
Dizziness, 101–105
Dupilumab, 123
Dysphagia, 157–160, **158**
Dysphonia, 141–144, **142**

E

EAC, *see* External auditory canal
Ear
behind the ear (BTE) hearing aid, 18
external ear trauma, 19–22
glue ear, 82
middle and inner ear structures, 15
outer ear (pinna) anatomy, 90
topical ear drops, 90, 91
Ear, nose and throat (ENT), 15, 19, 41, 55, 101, 111, 148
Endocrine screen, 127
ENT, *see* Ear, nose and throat
Epistaxis, 25–30
Epley manoeuvre, 105
External auditory canal (EAC), 82, 89, 90, 91, 97
External ear trauma, 19–22
External nasal anatomy, 41

F

Facial nerve, 15
Facial nerve palsy, 15, 17, 18, 111–116, 112, **113**
bilateral facial nerve palsy, 111
House-Brackmann scale for grading, **114**
Facial paralysis, 3
FB, *see* Foreign bodies
FESS, *see* Functional endoscopic sinus surgery
Flexible nasoendoscopy (FNE), 48, 53, 73, 76, 121,
126, 132, 142

Floseal/Surgicel, 29
FNE, *see* Flexible nasoendoscopy
Foley catheter, 28
FONA, *see* Front of neck access
Foreign bodies (FB), 61, 87
in upper aerodigestive tract, 61–64
Formal taste testing, 114
Free-field hearing tests, interpretation of, 82, **83**
Free-field testing, 81
Front of neck access (FONA), 50, 54
Functional endoscopic sinus surgery (FESS), 38, 123

G

Gentamicin, 91
Glue ear, 82
Gram-negative organisms, 89
Guillain-Barre syndrome, 111

H

Haematoma
orbital, 31–34, 32
pinna, 19, 22
post-thyroidectomy, 75–78, 76
septal, 41, 43
Haematomas
pinna, 19, 22
septal, 41, 43
Haemophilus influenzae, 3, 35
Head and neck, 45, 129
acute paediatric airway obstruction, 51–54
adult acute airway obstruction, 47–50, **48**
deep space neck infections, 65–69, **66**
dysphagia, 157–160, **158**
dysphonia, 141–144, **142**
head and neck malignancy, 131–136, **134**
malignancy of unknown primary, 137–140
neck trauma, 55–59, **56**, **57**
post-thyroidectomy haematoma, 75–78, 76
post-tonsillectomy bleed, 71–74, 72
salivary gland mass, 153–156
thyroid lump, 145–151, **146**
upper aerodigestive tract foreign body, 61–64
Head and neck malignancy, 131–136
TNM classification for, **134**
of unknown primary, 137
Head impulse test, 103
Hearing aids, 87
behind the ear (BTE) hearing aid, 18
contralateral routing of sound (CROS)
hearing aid, 18
Hearing loss, 15, 18
and audiology, 81–88, **82**
conductive hearing loss (CHL), 81, 85

Printed and bound by CPI Group (UK) Ltd, Croydon, CR0 4YY

17/10/2024

01775690-0003